Profit, Loss, and Miracles

Profit, Loss, and Miracles

Copyright © 2025 by Zelphoe Gabrielle Maloney and Robert Maloney

All rights reserved under the Pan-American and International Copyright Conventions. This book may not be reproduced in whole or in part, except for brief quotations embodied in critical articles or reviews, in any form or by any means, electronic or mechanical, including photocopying, recording, or by any information storage and retrieval system now known or hereinafter invented, without written permission of the publisher, Armin Lear Press.

ISBN (paperback): 978-1-963271-62-1
ISBN (eBook): 978-1-963271-63-8

Armin Lear Press, Inc.
215 W Riverside Drive, #4362
Estes Park, CO 80517

Profit, Loss, and *Miracles*

Zelphoe Gabrielle Maloney
& Robert Maloney

with thanks to Colonel Frank Borman

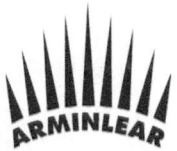
ARMINLEAR

Contents

1	Living at the Edge of Death	1
2	Surprises	11
3	Breakthrough to Hope—for Five Minutes	21
4	Overnight Denial	29
5	External Appeal	45
6	Unwelcome	61
7	A Shot in the Dark	67
8	Maloneys vs. Goliaths	73
9	The Lone Media Voice	85
10	A Powerful Ally	95
11	Betrayed	105
12	Sabotage	111
13	Adding Insult to Injury	117
14	Assaulted, and Again	123
15	A Promise of Hope	129
16	Reach for the Moon	137
17	Assassinations	149
18	Rebirth	155
19	Another Deal with the Devil	169
20	Firestorm	179
21	A Perfect Match	183
22	Scapegoating	193
23	New Hope	197
24	Whose Side Are You on, God?	211
25	Fire and Ice	217
26	The Price Tag on My Life	225
27	The Case of the Dubious Expert Witness	233
28	Unwavering Resolve	237
29	Stress	241
30	Forgiveness	245
Epilogue		249

One

Living at the Edge of Death

I was a young mother of five tethered to a tank of oxygen. If it hadn't been for my husband and children, I might have taken scissors to the thin leash connecting me to life.

By the end of 2003, the daily pain from my lupus made me worthless around our home; I thought my situation could not get any worse. But in the spring of 2004, I came to terms with my new normal and realized I had dropped to an even lower rung of hell. It's that place where you just know everyone who sees you either feels pity or revulsion.

Late on a sunny morning, after a sleepless night, I sat at the edge of my bed in my pajamas, listening to the sparrows play outside my window. Sometimes, consistent pain becomes part of who you are as your mind adapts and accepts its place in your life. But something as simple as a bird's song can briefly transport you to a blissful, pain-free state—better than good drugs because you're awake and aware.

The phone on the nightstand rang.

"Robert!" I called. I pushed myself into a sitting position and leaned toward the table, but I would not be able to reach the phone unless I stood up.

As I waited for Robert to answer the phone, I looked up and caught my reflection in the mirror above the dresser. By the time I took another tank-assisted breath, tears began to stream down my cheeks, dropping from my chin and soaking into my pajamas. *Where have I gone?* The woman my husband once called beautiful had been replaced by a withered, 90-pound skeleton who looked twice her age. The smooth face my husband had caressed with delight now resembled a rotting orange peel with a wig of straw. *What have I done to be punished this way?*

When despair settled in, however, the realization that others in the world were experiencing similar challenges brought back a sense of gratitude. *I'm still alive.* I took a moment to pray for the sick and homeless, most of whom didn't have the aroma of bacon wafting up the stairs from a modern kitchen.

Robert had answered the phone in the office, and I could hear him talking with a representative from Cigna, who was transferring ownership of our health insurance carrier, Lovelace, to Ardent. The thought of a trip to the bathroom caused me to tremble, and I debated whether to wait for Robert to finish his phone call and ask him for help. The bathroom was only a few feet away, but it might as well have been at the other end of town. The soles of my feet were so swollen I thought they might pop if they touched the floor.

I slowly slid my foot off the bed, leaving it dangling an inch from the floor. I looked up and inhaled deeply, then slowly let the breath escape my lips. I stretched my leg until my big toe reached the floor. Immediately, I jerked it up as pain seared through my body. I slammed my head back to the pillow and covered my mouth with my hand to keep from screaming.

Sucking down breaths, I took a moment to deal with the increased pain. I could hear Robert arguing with the Cigna representative. I rolled over onto my stomach as the tears flowed—this time from intense pain, not just anticipation of it. Using every ounce of strength in my arms to grip the sheets, I slowly slid down until my inflamed knees rested on the floor. I crawled, using my elbows to pull me forward like a six-month-old infant. But as I had seen five times before with my children, babies crawl with anticipation and wonder. I crawled with despair and disgust. Every shift of weight brought a sensation like nail-studded burning coals pressing into my knees as I strained to keep my toes from touching the floor. At the foot of the bed, I paused for a moment to suck in a few more breaths. When my strength gave way, and my toes pounded on the floor, I wailed. Everything went black.

Light engulfed me, and the pain was gone. I cannot describe the light because there is nothing from this life to compare it to, but it was beautiful. I gazed about as peace overtook my thoughts. Then complete darkness fell again. I was floating, but I could not see, hear, smell, or feel anything. I did not want my life to end like this. I started thinking about my husband and children.

Then I heard Robert crying, and the pain shot up my legs once again. It seems that a will to survive brings back all that life has to offer, from the face of love to the pain that robs you of joy.

Robert later described what happened after I collapsed during my journey to the bathroom. He heard my wails and ran through the hall, past the twins' bedroom, and into ours, where he saw me lying on my side, motionless. As he rushed in, he noticed the immense swelling of my feet. "Gabby!" he cried out and lifted me from the floor, cradling me in his arms.

Tears formed in his eyes as he looked up as if seeking an answer from heaven. After a few pounding beats of his heart, he closed his eyes, lowered his head, and sobbed.

Robert once told me, "Every other problem in the world seems microscopic when you're pondering how to tell your children that their mother has died." In his journal he wrote, *There are times in a man's life when he can accept failure. Losing his wife is not one of them.*

Perspective is a word he often uses when he explains how he felt during times like this. "I wished I could have traded places with you," he explained, "but then I think how unfair that would be. How could I ask you to watch me suffer?"

Lying in his arms, I moaned, rolled my eyes, and went limp. Robert quickly carried me out of the bedroom and down the hall, yelling to the nanny, "I've got to get her to the hospital! Take care of the kids."

She stepped out of the kitchen. "Oh my God! What happened?" she screamed as she raised her hands to her face and watched Robert carry me outside.

Robert belted me into the minivan and put it in gear. Tires squealed, and we raced to the hospital. As he tells it, his concern for me blended with anger as he remembered the circumstances that had led us to this point.

* * *

One night at dinner, my husband and I were discussing the realistic danger that intravenous immunoglobulin (IVIG) treatments would permanently affect my kidney function. We had started to wonder if Dr. Frank O'Sullivan, my rheumatologist, was being more responsive to the requests of the insurance company than to ours.

Four-year-old Dimitri pulled on my shirt and scowled: "Why do they want to kill your kidney?" My son's innocent question had teeth. Why would my doctor recommend a procedure that had been proven to damage kidney function? Should I take my child's innocent words as a dire warning? It reminded me of the scene in Shakespeare's *King Lear* when we see that Lear's wits are gone and there is a plot to kill him. The king and his loyal followers don't know who to trust anymore, and then the Fool blurts out: "He's mad that trusts in the tameness of a wolf."

I felt as though I was going mad—trying to trust wolves in white lab coats.

So much disappointment and fear had gone into creating this encroaching sense of insanity. Well, before this moment, I'd felt I was going mad looking for an answer to why everything that defined me as a woman was being taken away from me: intimacy with my husband, nurturing my children, a satisfying career, my physical appearance, and my connections with friends. So much had become out of reach for me, from the simple act of preparing a meal for people I love to the miracle of giving birth. Nothing on that broad spectrum was within my ability anymore. What good was I if I couldn't even make my children a sandwich?

As a little girl, I envisioned my fairytale life of professional success and a prince to share my life with. When I was twenty-one years old, I married my husband, Robert, a handsome student at a military academy. We planned to raise our children in an active lifestyle, with the whole family running, jumping, swimming, and eating healthy foods. I fueled the dream by running several miles each week and preparing nutritious meals at home. I pursued my degree in nursing and looked forward to applying to medical school. My dreams were coming true.

One day, I was procrastinating about walking on the treadmill when I received a call from my doctor's office—it was 1992. The doctor wanted to see me in his office the next morning. I didn't need the worried tone in the receptionist's voice to tell me something was wrong. At this point, I already knew I was falling short with my family—I couldn't properly get my children ready for school or bring myself to exercise. Instead of having a head full of dreams, I had a body overcome with fatigue. I didn't even have the energy to imagine a fairytale life, much less live one.

At ten o'clock the next morning, I walked into a waiting room of crying babies and agitated adults. The sound of my name rang through the air. I paced behind the closed door of the waiting room where a nurse had taken me. I could not take a full breath; even without seeing the doctor, my body went into a mild state of panic.

The door opened. "You have lupus," he said.

Medicine was my field; health was my passion. I knew the symptoms. I wasn't shocked. But knowing the facts about a disease and having the facts take hold of your life are two different experiences. I cried as I listened to a clinical explanation of how lupus is an autoimmune disease, a disease in which the immune system attacks its organs, just as it would attack an infection.

Without realizing it, I immediately started evolving into a textbook case for displaying the first four of Elisabeth Kübler-Ross's five stages of grief. But she was talking about the emotional experiences of terminally ill patients—how they went through denial, anger, bargaining, depression, and finally acceptance. I knew no matter how angry or depressed I got, I would never accept lupus as a death sentence—never.

My initial thought was a declaration of denial: *This will go away like a bad cold.* Then I told myself, *The doctor can manage it with little impact on my ability to live as I wish.* The problem was that most doctors knew little about lupus or how to treat it, so I was told I needed a rheumatologist.

The nurse took me to another waiting area, which was almost as packed as the waiting room in the lobby. People stared at me as tears ran down my cheeks. Nurses walked by, continuing with their business, while I waited for a referral to a specialist. The next thing I remember, I was home. How I got there is a complete blank, but apparently, I made it on my own.

Within months, the lupus had attacked every organ in my body, from my skin to my brain. We raced to the emergency room countless times. By this point, I felt I had little choice but to surrender control of my health to physicians. Doctors told me to limit my exposure to sunlight, so even sitting comfortably in a chair with the afternoon light on me was suddenly a health hazard. They prescribed steroids in an attempt to control the swelling of my organs and joints. My beloved Robert went into protection mode.

He did everything the doctors asked and limited my activities in an attempt to shield me from pain. Looking back, I realize he was scared. Was he afraid of losing me, afraid the doctors would make a mistake, afraid our children would grow up without their mother, or perhaps afraid of something he didn't understand? All I know is that he pushed through the fear, slowly transforming his fear into hope.

Neither one of us would venture anywhere near Kübler-Ross's final stage of acceptance.

For years, I was sick for almost every event in my life. I would call Robert home early from work to attend the kids' school plays and sports games in my place. Sometimes, it was because I felt physically exhausted, and sometimes, I was so embarrassed by my deformed appearance, caused by inflammation and long-term steroid use, that I chose to remain at home, fighting my depression. This lack of participation fueled the guilt I felt over my family's daily worry about me, and I often wondered if the burden of my care was becoming too much for them. Instead of preparing meals for my children, I lay in bed while my children prepared meals and brought them to their helpless, listless mothers. Sometimes, that was the only time I saw my children during the day.

Lupus had turned me into a lonely woman.

And a fearful one. As lupus kept attacking parts of my body, I had this image that it was some amorphous shape that would invade my organs and, as part of wreaking havoc on them, would take away life and leave behind fear. Day after day, I became more afraid of what might happen next. From the beginning of my diagnosis, doctors told me my kidneys were compromised, and my fear increased the more I understood the consequences of kidney failure. I would stay home and cry at the thought that something as simple as sitting in the sun to watch my children play soccer could trigger a lupus flare. Every flare would result in my immune system killing a portion of my kidneys or damaging one or more of my other organs.

Sometimes, I tried to hide the pain so I could attend a wedding or holiday dinner, but this usually resulted in a hospital stay. The physical pain that accompanied borderline mass organ failure put me into a nightmarish mental state; having doctors and nurses tending to me around the clock was, ironically, more disconcerting than comforting. Off and on for eighteen of thirty-six months, I was confined to a bed in that same hospital. If not for the daily visits from my husband, I would have been the most lonely and afraid woman on the planet—or so I often thought.

But sometimes, when I was alone, I pictured myself at the beach with my family. I imagined the smell of the ocean and laughing as our children played in the surf. I listened to the crash of the waves as they rolled in and got louder as the tide came in. It was thoughts like these, thoughts of being normal again, that gave my will to survive just enough lift to sustain me another day.

Robert and I clutched at hope with everything we had. We expected at least some kind of positive attitude and team spirit from the healthcare professionals around us.

Two

Surprises

I knew I had a serious problem the day after a car accident that occurred on my way home from college in 1992. I was a married mother of two who worked weekends and attended classes on Tuesdays and Thursdays. The accident seemed minor, but shortly after the collision, my body started doing abnormal things. At the time, I couldn't be precise about what was different, though, and convincing my doctor that something was wrong would take months.

I was rear-ended on I-40 at the Eubank exit in Albuquerque. I sustained minor injuries, which seemed superficial at the time. At most, I may have suffered a bit of whiplash. But when I awoke the next day, I felt confused and disoriented.

"You should see a doctor," Robert insisted as he headed off to work.

"I'll try to get in today," I said automatically, although I was unsure why I needed to see the doctor.

Two days later, Robert left work early and took me to the doctor, as I had not gone on my own. I wasn't trying to be stubborn. I was scared because, within these two days, I had begun to unexpectedly forget where I was. Without realizing it, I had even walked into my neighbor's house.

"What are you doing?" she asked.

She looked familiar, but I couldn't place her. I froze. As she approached me, I raised my arms to keep her away and started to cry.

"It's okay," she said in a calm voice.

"I don't know where I am," I explained.

She put her arm around me and helped me to my apartment. I remained confused until Robert opened the door. Crying, I ran past him and into our bedroom.

"I'm sorry," Robert was saying to the neighbor. "I'll take her in to be checked out."

At that moment, my memory of my neighbor Donna suddenly clicked in my mind. I wondered what was wrong with me, that suddenly my memory had an on-and-off switch. This is when Robert took me to our general practitioner.

The doctor ruled out a concussion and whiplash but did not have an answer for what was causing my confusion spells. Due to the rapid onset of periods of disorientation, within two weeks, I had to drop out of college.

Besides memory loss, dizzy spells, and nausea, I developed severe joint pain, including back and neck stiffness, semicircle rashes on my body, and a butterfly rash on my cheeks. I wanted to be referred to a chiropractor. Still, my doctor reminded me that my husband's work health plan did not cover chiropractic services, and the symptoms I was experiencing were common after an accident. I decided to get a second opinion and then a third. None of the doctors could figure out what was causing my symptoms. Eventually my husband made arrangements for me to see a chiropractor under my auto insurance policy's personal injury provision.

On my first visit, the chiropractor made mild adjustments that relieved some of the stiffness and pain. He examined the rashes and said, "I've seen this before, especially in Hispanic females." He looked more closely. "But if it's what I think it is, it can affect anyone. I have other patients with similar symptoms. We need to ask your doctor to run some specific tests."

What had the other doctors missed?

A few weeks after the lab tests, I received a call from my doctor's office. The results confirmed the chiropractor's suspicion of lupus. It was June of 1992 and the beginning of my intimate experience of for-profit health care. Or, as my husband would say, "It was when a price tag was put on your life."

I started the standard first line of treatment, an anabolic steroid called prednisone. Anabolic steroids are drugs related to male sex hormones, and that's why they are banned, performance-enhancing substances in amateur (and most professional) athletics. They promote the growth of skeletal muscle, so for a person with lupus or HIV, for example, they are used to counter the kind of wasting of the body associated with those diseases. But to be clear, prednisone is not one of the bodybuilder types of anabolic steroids. It's designed to prevent the release of inflammation-causing substances in the body, not to make you look like Arnold Schwarzenegger. It also suppresses the immune system.

And then there are the hideous side effects. All of them don't happen to everyone, but since I was already beating the odds by getting a disease that only affects less than ½ of one percent of the population, I was bound to score high on the side-effects scale, wasn't I? The litany includes confusion (as though I wasn't already confused with lupus), excitement, restlessness, headache, nausea, vomiting, thinning skin, trouble sleeping, weight gain, skin rash, depression—you get the picture.

The good news was that the co-payment for my prednisone was just five dollars. As a couple in the early 1990s who could barely afford the $280-per-month family-plan insurance premiums through Borden, the cost was attractive.

Looking back, Robert and I both wish we had asked more questions. Robert trusted the medical profession, and I was in denial (Kübler-Ross was so right about this one.) I kept telling myself, "I'm only in my twenties, I eat well, and I exercise. This will go away soon." Our trust in healthcare professionals, as well as our young age, left us exposed to insurance company bureaucracy. Suppose we had educated ourselves on the side effects of steroids and researched alternative treatments. In that case, the next five years of physical and mental hell I endured might have been eliminated or at least minimized.

It was only a few months after beginning the steroid regimen that I experienced increased weight gain. At first, I cut back on eating and exercised as much as the pain allowed. Then I had to buy new clothes. This was devastating for a woman who had never been above a size 4. Soon, I was deformed beyond recognition, almost twice my usual weight. I had gained close to 80 pounds, and my new body fat was distributed disproportionately. My face looked as if it was swollen from a beating, a condition called "moon face." Balls of fat formed under my arms and under the back of my neck, to the point that I appeared to have a hunchback. People I hadn't seen in months didn't recognize me. When the swelling was severe, my children were afraid to get close to me. I was hideous, not from the lupus alone, but from the side effects of the prednisone.

For the five years that I was on this steroid regimen, I complained of the side effects to my doctor—and for five years, nothing changed. What did change, however, was my self-esteem. It plunged below zero. On some scale, you can relate if you were ever a teenager. Your skin isn't perfect, your weight isn't perfect, the "right" person in high school doesn't know you exist, a cool kid bullies you, you didn't make the team you wanted, you don't get invited to any parties, and/or you were told in auditions for the school musical that you can't sing a note. In short, you feel like suicide is a happy alternative to the life you now have. Now multiply that by ten because you're a helpless, worthless mother whose children don't recognize you, and you feel like a kiss goodnight from your husband is an act of charity.

My insecurity weighed heavily on my marriage, and my social life shrank to nothing. I was embarrassed to be out in public and sought any opportunity to remain at home. Every time Robert communicated with women for any reason, I doubted my womanhood, and my heart filled with the fear that I was no longer attractive.

Robert had always told me, "I only have eyes for you," and I believed him. A poem he wrote for me during this time still adorns the wall of my bedroom, framed with pictures he chose to remind me of his love.

The Color of Love

You ask me what's my favorite
But that is hard to say.
You ask me what's my favorite
But it changes every day.
Could it be the color brown, or pink, or maybe red?
I can't decide on one of these, they're always in my head.
Could it be the color brown, the color of your eyes?
In my mind I think of them, and then my heart it flies.
Could it be the color pink, the color of your lips?
They are sweet as sweet as wine, and I cherish every sip.
Could it be the color red? Your hair is what I see
Oh so shiny and so soft, as soft as it could be.
You ask me what's my favorite,
That is hard to do
But if I had to choose right now
I'd choose the color YOU.

But knowing he loved me was not the same as feeling that I deserved his loving gaze. Robert and I were in our twenties, and it felt as if my condition had robbed us of our youth. He never complained, but certain things he loved to do, like going out on dates with me, coaching our children's sports teams, hunting, and fishing with our children, fell by the wayside. When you look in the mirror and something unrecognizable looks back, it takes its toll. Ultimately, my guilt over being sick was superseded by my pain and deformity. In movies like *Love Story*, the female lead looks pale and weak but never ugly. Jenny Cavalleri (actress Ali MacGraw) dies, but she remains beautiful to the end.

I remember that I later discovered from a nurse friend that prescribing steroids is the preferred first option for insurance companies because it is the least expensive alternative. If you're a number-cruncher, that makes sense. If you're a healthcare provider, how could it make sense?

Steroids do relieve some of the inflammation but do nothing to cure lupus itself. On its website, the Mayo Clinic describes the benefits and risks in these terms: "Corticosteroids can counter the inflammation of lupus but often produce long-term side effects—including weight gain, easy bruising, thinning bones (osteoporosis), high blood pressure, diabetes and increased risk of infection. The risk of side effects increases with higher doses and longer term therapy." I still had constant lupus flares and was hospitalized due to organ and bone damage. I eventually developed osteopenia (low bone density) and osteonecrosis (dead bone). Those five years of mental anguish ripped at both my marriage and my sanity. And for what?

This is both the truth and harsh reality that you, or someone you love, probably have experienced: The insurance company could save money by treating the symptoms instead of the cause.

At this point, you might be saying, "Yeah. That's what they do."

But I fought back. Robert and I fought back. We kept punching and ultimately thought we had them on the mat.

After researching the options, my husband and I demanded alternative treatments. To our surprise, we met with little resistance from our doctor. In fact, he almost seemed relieved by our decision. Based on my experience, I've concluded that insurance companies dictate the order of options to doctors, who must follow them. The doctors understand the risks and dangers these options present but are limited in suggesting other treatments unless we, as patients, get specific and deliberate in our requests.

Over the next few years, I regained not only my normal weight but also my social life and resumed a healthy relationship with my husband. But the alternatives to steroids had their side effects. A medication like Imuran (generic: azathioprine) is an immunosuppressant, so it weakens the body's immune system. The side effects of long-term use include an increased risk of getting certain types of cancers, blood disorders, and stomach problems. With Imuran, I got the benefit of controlling my lupus symptoms, but I also had adverse effects on appetite and digestion. The occasional diarrhea and fatigue were welcome alternatives to the mental anguish steroids had caused. Plaquenil also helped, but it did not eliminate the lupus flares. Plaquenil (generic: hydroxychloroquine sulfate) is an interesting drug used to both prevent and treat malaria infections caused by mosquito bites. In conjunction with other medications, though, it's used to treat autoimmune diseases like lupus—but only when other medications either have not worked or can't be tolerated by the patient. Most of the side effects won't surprise you: the usual nausea, stomach cramps, loss of appetite, diarrhea, dizziness, and headaches. There was one potential side effect of this that really frightened me, though. Plaquenil can cause serious, permanent eye damage. Ever since I got the lupus diagnosis, my biggest fears were that I would lose my kidneys and/or my sight. The relief from symptoms seemed worth the risk.

During this time of non-steroid use, I had several lupus flares and was hospitalized multiple times as the effectiveness of the alternative medications diminished. Eventually none of the conventional methods worked. Still, I was grateful for the temporary relief that these drugs provided.

What I really needed was a medical miracle.

Three

Breakthrough to Hope—for Five Minutes

It was now 2003, more than ten years since I had been diagnosed. The experience had taken its toll on my body and will to survive. Hospitalization happened every few weeks, and every possible treatment we knew of had been tried with only temporary and limited success. It seemed that cyclophosphamide was the only remaining option, even though I had tried it before with negative results.

It was five years earlier, in 1998, when my rheumatologist-of-the-moment ordered cycles of cyclophosphamide. Robert and a close friend accompanied me to the hospital that morning. I was terrified of the possible side effects of getting this injected into me because I had researched the side effects on the Mayo Clinic website: "swelling of feet or lower legs, unusual tiredness or weakness, sores in the mouth and lips, sudden shortness of breath, nausea or vomiting, diarrhea, swollen lips, and stomach pain."

As I remember, the nurse escorted us into the outpatient services room and asked me to remove my jacket. When she returned with the IV bag of cyclophosphamide, she handed me a small cup that contained a pill. "You'll need to take that," she said. "It will help with the nausea."

Robert poured me a cup of water from the little pink pitcher on the bedside table, saying, "Don't worry, hon. This won't take long."

The nurse inserted the needle in my arm and connected the IV tube. "I'll start with a slow drip and will increase it after we see how you're doing," she explained. She adjusted the drip and left the room.

My friend started talking to Robert and me about finalizing her divorce. Suddenly, I couldn't breathe. I looked at Robert and slammed my hand on the bed, trying to speak.

Robert stood up. "What's wrong?"

"Quick, call the nurse!" my friend shouted.

I started shaking my head as I gasped for air.

Robert pushed the nurse button and ran out of the room, shouting, "Nurse, nurse!"

The voice of the nurse came over the intercom, "How can I help you?"

My friend yelled, "She can't breathe!"

The nurse ran in, holding a needle, with Robert following close behind. She closed off the drip and inserted the needle into the IV tube.

"What the hell is happening?" Robert demanded.

I regained my ability to breathe as the nurse slowly forced the liquid into the IV tube.

"I'm sorry, Mr. Maloney," she said. "I believe she reacted to the cyclophosphamide, but we need the doctor to confirm. The Benadryl® is kicking in. She'll be all right."

I reached for Robert's hand as I inhaled precious air. Benadryl is a wonder drug for some people. A friend who had to go through several rounds of chemotherapy for cancer had a nurse drip Benadryl into her IV lines to prevent any allergic reaction—like the one I'd had to cyclophosphamide. She breezed through the five-hour chemo sessions, breathing easily and sleeping well thanks to the medication.

A few years later, a friend in the medical field suggested a possible reason for my reaction. In some cases, there are differences in the tolerability of cyclophosphamide regimens. Apparently, the price difference between various cyclophosphamide regimens might have played a role in my reaction to the drug. In other words, there can be quality differences between cyclophosphamide regimens.

I made my rheumatologist, Dr. O'Sullivan, aware of my reaction to cyclophosphamide, and he opted to prescribe a high dose of CellCept, a drug used as an anti-rejection medication for transplant patients. At first, he prescribed 1,000 mg, but after a few months, he increased it to 1,500 mg and finally 2,500 mg. My body's reaction to the 2,500 mg daily dose included uncontrollable diarrhea and dehydration. My weight dropped to less than 90 pounds, and I experienced severe and chronic fatigue, along with accidents, because I could not reach a bathroom in time. The CellCept was controlling my lupus, but in the process, I felt like it was killing me. My doctor's recommendation was to rest and drink PediaSure for nutrition. I was alive, but I was not living.

The need for my husband to look after me led him to cut back on his time at work. He reorganized and renamed our small business so he could spend more time caring for me. It was this change that revealed to us the unconscionable nature of the health insurance industry.

I remember in April 2003, Robert took me to O'Sullivan's office for a routine visit. He was a tall, thin man in his early fifties with graying blond hair, dressed in a lab coat, tie, and glasses that hung around his neck. He carried my very thick stack of medical records in his arms.

"How are the Maloneys today?" he asked.

Robert shook his hand and replied, "Gabrielle's condition is getting worse. It seems we're in urgent care every other week. Increasing her medications isn't cutting it."

O'Sullivan looked at my chart as Robert sat beside me and placed his hand in mine. I squeezed it and forced a smile.

The doctor looked up from the chart. "Well, it looks like Gabrielle's creatinine level is questionable. It's not good, but it's stable." Creatinine is a waste molecule transported through the bloodstream to the kidneys. If the kidneys are working properly, they filter it out, and then it's taken away in urine. He perked up a bit: "Were you able to get your new insurance? I see from my notes last month that you're changing plans."

Robert nodded. "Everything's changed over now."

The doctor asked me to sit on the exam table. After a routine exam, he asked Robert to help me back to the chair. "Besides weight loss, are there any new symptoms?" he asked.

After a weak cough, I replied, "The CellCept is really affecting me. I'm not sure what's worse, the pain or the side effects."

"Her weight has dropped dramatically," Robert interjected. "Everything passes right through her." I nodded in agreement.

At this point, I felt hopeless. All I expected to hear was, *We'll take more blood work, and I'll see you in two weeks.* Robert continued holding my hand, seemingly anticipating the same response.

His grip slowly tightened as O'Sullivan spoke. "I know a colleague who is working on clinical trials using stem cells to replace the immune system of lupus patients. I haven't spoken to her for almost a year, but I've been keeping up with the results of the study she's involved in through a medical journal. It might be our only alternative at this point."

I wasn't sure what to think, and by the look on Robert's face, he was just as confused. I had been close to death for the past two years, and just two weeks prior to our appointment, O'Sullivan said I might have only six months to live. Now, he was telling us of a potential cure he had known about for a year or longer. *Why now?* I wondered. *What changed? Why didn't you tell us about this earlier?* These questions should have exploded through our minds, but when you're this close to death, some questions, like *why*, seem irrelevant compared to others, like *when*.

Robert and I were at a loss for words. I finally had to let go of his hand, as he was hurting me with the pressure of his squeeze.

"It's called a stem cell transplant," he continued, "and I believe Dr. Traynor is having good success with it. I need to check again to make sure she's still conducting the transplants at Northwestern in Chicago. Let me make a note in your chart and see what I can find. I'll be back in a minute."

Robert seemed ecstatic, but I had reservations. I had heard this before. The chemotherapy was supposed to put my lupus into remission. *I will not submit so easily this time*, I thought, and then a tranquil feeling embraced me as I listened to Robert's optimistic words. A cinder of hope had been rekindled.

O'Sullivan returned and said, "All right. I've updated your chart and will type a referral for Dr. Traynor. She's transferred to UMass in Boston, but according to the journal, she's still actively participating in stem cell transplants. I'll contact her to make sure you qualify as a candidate. My nurse will call you as soon as I find out for sure. It's fairly new for treating lupus, but . . . the results do look promising."

The smile on Robert's face said more than any words he could have spoken, and for an instant, I believed as I uttered, "At this point, I'll try anything. My kids hardly see me except in bed."

"I know," O'Sullivan said, "but on a positive note, Blue Cross Blue Shield should cover the treatment."

Robert's eyes opened wide. "We don't have Blue Cross Blue Shield."

With a puzzled stare, the doctor said, "I thought you just switched last month."

"We did! When I closed one business and opened another, I dropped the Lovelace plan we had and started another Lovelace plan to take its place. That's the reason for the thirty-day lapse in coverage."

O'Sullivan leaned back against the exam table. "I thought you told me you were switching to Blue Cross Blue Shield."

"I would, but the Albuquerque Chamber of Commerce doesn't offer it."

My anxiety rose as the doctor's posture seemed to freeze.

Robert's tone shifted. "That doesn't matter, does it?"

O'Sullivan frowned. "Lovelace won't cover the treatment until all other possibilities are exhausted," he said.

Robert stood up and took a step toward him. "What other options? I thought you said it was our only viable treatment."

The absurdity of this conversation overwhelmed me. Before the promise of a possible treatment could even penetrate my thoughts, it had been ripped from me. I could tell the doctor's response made Robert angry. He tried to project optimism as the doctor continued, but he was seething.

"Lovelace will not even consider an out-of-network procedure until all possible in-network procedures are exhausted. I hate to say it, but an IVIG treatment given through an IV drip in an outpatient setting will have to be the next step. It would have to be monitored closely, as it could cause further kidney damage."

Reluctantly, we agreed to try the IVIG so that Lovelace would have no reason to disapprove of the stem cell transplant. O'Sullivan recommended the IVIG treatment to Lovelace, but at the same time, he sent in an approval request to Lovelace for Ann Traynor to do the stem cell transplant.

This is what we were discussing at dinner the night Dimitri pulled on my skirt and asked me why the doctor wanted to kill my kidney.

The referral for the stem cell transplant fell by the wayside as I prepared for the IVIG treatments that would begin on May 2, 2003. At first, the treatment, given over several days, felt like poison being forced through my veins. I had nausea and got an awful taste in my mouth, even though it was given through an IV. My blood work results of May 5 note, "Major difficulty with HTN [hypertension, or high blood pressure] after IVIG. Creatinine skyrockets." By my next appointment on May 9, I needed a wheelchair. I could not even use it myself. Robert had to push me everywhere I needed to go.

In response to this, O'Sullivan ordered lower doses spread out over a longer period. But the kidney damage continued. I learned that kidney failure would actually benefit the insurance company because, after one year on dialysis, the company could shift a patient to Medicare. This wouldn't have even occurred to me if one of the nurses hadn't mentioned it as a possibility. Shifting me to Medicare would release Lovelace from further expenses. It was not that Cytoxan or IVIG treatments in and of themselves were bad, but my nurse told me that Lovelace was only allowing the lowest quality of medications in an attempt to cut costs.

The procedure our doctor would have never proposed had been forced on us. After the failed IVIG treatment, I was given another treatment that had already failed me: Cytoxan. After several doses with no results, O'Sullivan stopped the treatments.

Four

Overnight Denial

With the IVIG treatments, the pain seemed to crawl to the surface from inside my body. They also obliterated my kidney; I was dying. O'Sullivan sent another request for a stem cell transplant to Lovelace and made it clear that we had, in fact, tried everything else. We wondered if Lovelace would finally approve the stem cell transplant or if their executives would just get annoyed that I was still holding on to life almost a year later after the initial request.

I was lying in bed watching television while Robert prepared dinner. It was six o'clock on a quiet spring evening on May 16, 2004. Veronica answered the phone and said, "Dad, telephone. Someone from Cigna."

A few moments later, Robert hurried excitedly into the bedroom, phone in hand, and sat on the bed next to me. "Hold on, please. I'm putting you on speaker." Robert held my hand. "Sir, could you repeat that?" he asked. I had no idea what was going on, but my anticipation peaked.

"Yes, Mr. Maloney," said the man on the phone. "The stem cell transplant has been approved. I will e-mail you a list of approved providers."

I covered my mouth with my hand, let out a deep breath, and began to cry.

"One more thing," the man said. "You need to make arrangements for your stay. Lovelace provides up to ten thousand dollars for expenses, including travel and lodging. I'll send you the list right now."

Robert let go of my hand and stood up. "Thank you, Mr. Coppola."

"It's my pleasure. Let me give you my number. Call me as soon as you decide on the location you choose for the transplant."

Robert took the phone off speaker, leaned over the nightstand, and began writing. "Thank you again," Robert said and set the phone down. He bent over and hugged me as tears rolled down his face. "You're going to make it," he said.

Robert was concerned about getting me to the treatment center as soon as possible, while I worried about who would look after the children. Robert sat by my side as I explained to my mother on the phone the need for her assistance in caring for the children over the next four months. She agreed, and I focused on all the things I knew she would need to care for the children. I also made a list of things for Robert to prepare.

The next morning, on May 17, while Robert and I were still in bed, the phone rang again. Robert took the phone out of the bedroom. A few moments later, I heard him yelling, "You told us yesterday that it was approved and we were going to have ten thousand dollars available to cover expenses. What happened to 'Don't worry, all you need to do is pick the hospital and pack?' How do you expect me to tell my wife it's been denied? Let me speak with your supervisor!"

I prayed I was dreaming. I can't describe the horror I felt as those words came crashing down: "It's been denied." Tears began to stream down my cheeks as I sat motionless and listened to the continuing conversation.

"What kind of insensitive bastard is this, Dan, to tell me my wife's procedure is denied? I don't ever want to speak to that son of a bitch again! He told us just yesterday it was approved! What the fuck is going on?"

I waited. I'm not sure what I was waiting for, maybe a kiss on the cheek from Robert to wake me so we could plan the trip, or even the face of Jesus calling me home. All I know is I waited.

Robert yelled again, "An appeal? Are you kidding me? My wife is dying!" His voice faded as I heard the front door open and close, just like my chance for survival.

Robert's anger was immediate and intense. Mine took weeks to set in; once again, I plunged straight into denial.

When Robert returned, he walked into our room and looked at my face. He knew I had heard. He hugged me and whispered, "They have to give you a chance. They cannot approve something and then take it away. It's not right."

"What do we do?" I asked.

Robert sighed. "I'll file an appeal, and we just have to wait."

"I don't have much time," I whispered back. Robert tightened his hug.

Days dragged on as we waited for an official denial to be mailed to us. Nothing else seemed to matter, and all we could do was speculate about what was happening behind the scenes after we faxed our appeal back to Cigna. After additional phone calls, Robert believed that the appeal was approved, and the representative was making sure before she sent us a confirmation of approval to avoid a repeat of the first fiasco. Meanwhile, I was afraid to hope for anything. According to my attorney's notes about the facts surrounding the approval/denial discovered in testimony, this is what transpired among Lovelace, Cigna, and us on May 17, 2004:

> 5/17/04 8:20 a.m. (MST) Dan Coppola notifies UMass that Zelphoe Maloney is denied treatment for bone marrow transplant.
>
> 5/17/04 9:19 a.m. (MST) Dan Coppola notes: Forward denial request to Dr. Sunderman (Lovelace's medical director).
>
> 5/17/04 10:00 a.m. (MST) Zelphoe receives notice over the phone that insurance denied request.
>
> 5/17/04 10:47 a.m. (MST) Dan Coppola actually faxes denial request form to Dr. Sunderman for review and signature.
>
> 5/17/04 10:54 a.m. (MST) Denial signed by Sunderman, apparently in minutes, with no detail given

by Sunderman. According to Kim Livingston, this would appear to be the first activity on the file by Albuquerque Lovelace. Livingston picks up signed denial from Sunderman. She fills out "denial letter request form" that says in cross-hatched area that's mostly illegible "Phone notification" (blank), "Person Notified" (blank), and "Option to discuss with medical director" (N/A).

5/17/04 2:17 p.m. (MST) Notice of denial faxed to Maloney.

5/17/04 3:04 p.m. (MST) Maloney faxes back completed official appeal form.

The anomalies in those notes become clear, and take center stage when our battle with Lovelace escalated in the coming years.

During the time we waited for an answer to our request, Robert and I discussed what we needed to take care of before we left to receive my transplant. Just then, his phone rang. After listening for a moment, he stood up and left the room, the phone to his ear.

A few minutes later, he returned, wrapped his arms around me, and said, "The stem cell transplant is denied. I'll fax back a request for an internal appeal."

I sank into a pit of hopelessness, overwhelmed by the constant pain, the fact I weighed less than 90 pounds, the fatigue that ruled my days, and the reality that my youngest children were afraid to come close to me because of my deformed face.

* * *

Lovelace was required to respond to our appeal request within ten days or obtain an additional ten days if needed. On Thursday, June 3, 2004, seventeen days after we filed our appeal, Robert again called Cigna to see why we had not received a determination of our request for an internal appeal. He was put on hold several times, and his call was transferred to multiple representatives. Finally, the supervisor who had asked Robert to submit the appeal came on the line and said she would need to call us back.

The call never came. On Wednesday, June 9, we received a denial letter dated June 4. Joel Newton, who would eventually represent us, describes the incident like this in his letter to Madison, Harbour & Mroz, PA, attorneys for Cigna:

> Two days after the denial of the bone marrow transplant (BMT) on that Monday, May 17, one of the world's leading experts in BMT for lupus wrote the subcontractor (Cigna) asking for an "expedited appeal" (which has a 72-hour appeal deadline). That BMT world expert sent several peer-reviewed articles supporting BMT as safe and highly effective. The subcontractor called to report the letter and articles. Lovelace said that it wasn't interested in having the articles sent to them . . . That subcontractor nurse said in his adjuster's diary entries that Lovelace was "treating this as an expedited appeal," but Lovelace did not respond until June 4, 2004 (13 business days after the denial). Lovelace had 72 hours for this life-and-death decision if it truly was treating it as "expedited," but it apparently lost the packet in its offices.

Even if Lovelace did not treat this as an "expedited appeal," Lovelace sent the Maloneys a letter saying how long they had under standard appeal deadlines. It told them it was required to rule on Mrs. Maloney's appeal of the BMT denial "within ten days"—by May 31, 2004. Robert Maloney called Lovelace every day from May 31 until June 4, finally getting someone at Lovelace to pay attention to him.

By the way, his poor wife had lost 25 pounds in the previous 30 days, and he was having to carry her in and out of the shower, to doctor's office visits, and to and from bed. He had to toilet her. She was dying right before his very eyes. Her pain score remained a constant 8:10 or above, day and night. So Robert Maloney called again and again.

The appeals representative who finally answered Robert said that at 11:07 Robert called. That appeals rep went and "found the packet," assembled the additional information needed for it, put it in front of the medical director doing this "Tier I" review, and a denial decision was made by 12:00 (about 45 minutes after Robert called—just in time for the medical director's lunch).

On Thursday, June 10, 2004, Robert filed an expedited request for an internal panel review.

When you read Joel's recap of the events with Lovelace, you were probably thinking of all the times insurance companies did things to you that made no sense. For years, stories like this from other people have kept my head spinning. The near-nonsensical nature of the Lovelace employees' responses made me think of how baffled Alice was when she ended up at the Mad Hatter's tea party: "The Hatter's remark seem to have no sort of meaning in it, and yet it was certainly English." (from Lewis Carroll's *Alice's Adventures in Wonderland*)

Unfortunately, the nonsense was just beginning.

After the first denial, I asked O'Sullivan for a letter stating the medical necessity of the stem cell transplant for my survival as evidence for the internal appeal board. He wrote a letter to Lovelace on my behalf on June 11, 2004.

> This is a respectful request of appeal related to your denial of coverage for an autologous hematopoietic stem cell transplant . . . for a patient who has severe and refractory lupus nephritis. The patient has been under my care since November of 2001. She was given the diagnosis of systemic lupus erythematosus approximately ten or 11 years ago . . . I have attempted to treat her lupus nephritis with essentially all available immunosuppressive therapies, including high-dose corticosteroids, Imuran, Cytoxan, high-dose intravenous immunoglobulin, and CellCept. In spite of these efforts, the patient's renal function has continued to deteriorate. Autologous stem cell transplantation has been shown to be a significant beneficial treatment, which salvages

renal function in patients with refractory lupus nephritis.

We have referred the patient to a transplant center, the University of Massachusetts, where the transplant program is directed by one of the nation's leading experts in stem cell transplantation for autoimmune disease, Dr. Ann Traynor. It is my expert opinion as a board certified specialist in the treatment of systemic lupus erythematosus that if the patient remains on her current therapy, she will experience inevitable progression to end stage renal failure . . . Autologous stem cell transplantation offers the only possible hope of avoiding this outcome. I urge you to reconsider your denial to cover this procedure, which will provide Mrs. Maloney with an opportunity to lead a normal life.

My father often said, "Haste is the companion of deceit." I heard his words in my head just before our internal appeal hearing with the insurance company.

Robert and I, along with the regional trainer, were hosting an education session for the store managers of our business on Thursday, June 17, 2004, at 12:30 p.m. The meeting was about to begin when Robert took a call. After a few minutes, he excused himself and asked the trainer and me to follow him. Robert was visibly upset, and I had no clue what was going on. Then he asked the trainer if she could drive us to a meeting across town. We had carpooled with her so we could discuss the agenda for the meeting, and our car was at another location.

Disbelief and confusion combined as Robert repeated what the Lovelace representative had said: "Your internal appeal hearing is in thirty minutes. Do you plan to attend?" I could feel my blood pressure rising as Robert rushed us to the car, and by the time we reached Lovelace's corporate office, my vision was beginning to blur.

The three people seated around the table ignored us when we entered. They continued talking among themselves as they pushed piles of paper from one person to another. The look of compassion Robert wore as he helped me sit down immediately shifted as he turned to face the panel.

"How dare you?" he shouted. "We had no advance notice of this meeting. I had to leave another meeting on the other side of town to get here in less than thirty minutes. I would have brought the letter of medical necessity from Dr. O'Sullivan if I had known." As Robert paused to catch his breath, I looked at the stunned panel. Robert pointed in turn at every panel member. "My wife is dying. And this is the way you treat her? I can't believe you did this!" He slammed his fist on the table. "Look at her! Look at her!"

At that moment, I realized it was time *I* got angry. But I wasn't sure who should be the target of my anger—the people seated at the table or some nameless, faceless person in a huge office overlooking the ocean hundreds of miles from Albuquerque.

After the meeting, Robert looked up the procedure stated in Lovelace's member handbook that was supposed to be followed for this appeal meeting. In essence, what they had done was like changing the rules of the game after the first quarter was already underway.

> Unless you choose not to pursue your appeal, we will notify you of the date, time and place of the Medical Panel Review . . . No fewer than (3) working days prior to the Medical Panel Review, we will provide to you the following information: your pertinent medical records; your treatment provider's recommendation; the summary of benefits for your health benefit plan; a copy of notice of the adverse determination; generally accepted practice guidelines, evidence-based practice guidelines or practice guidelines developed by the federal government or national and professional medical societies, boards and associations; any applicable clinical review criteria, policies or protocols used by us in making the adverse determination; and all other evidence or documentation relevant in reviewing the adverse determination.

The process we had just experienced bore no resemblance to that description.

The panel was composed of two Lovelace physicians who had never seen me as a patient or a person before. The entire appeal hearing took less than thirty minutes. Each member asked me questions about failed treatments I had received and if I had thoroughly researched the stem cell transplant I requested. Robert demanded that the letter of medical necessity be added to the file. One panel member agreed to request a copy of the file. Only one panel member—the non-Lovelace person—seemed moved by my pleas for a chance at life.

Abruptly, the panel stood up, and the person at the end of the table said, "We'll have a determination within forty-eight hours."

Joel Newton's breakdown of the internal appeal explains the fight we were in with our hands tied behind our backs. The parenthetical comments spotlight anomalies and egregious errors.

> The Maloneys appealed the Tier I denial to what is called a Tier II panel. The Tier II panel must be composed of a specialist medical director who currently practices handling these types of cases (Lovelace had no such specialist on the panel).
>
> Lovelace also promises a "non-Lovelace physician" on the panel. Dr. Berman, the doctor chosen, was a retired allergist, a 30-plus-year former Lovelace employee ... Dr. Berman was retired (not up on new technology even if had he practiced in this area). As a 30-year retiree from Lovelace who made extra money by serving regularly on these panels, he hardly fit the "non-Lovelace" requirement, either. By regulation, Lovelace had to provide the Maloneys and the panel with "uniform standards" (the guidelines for the decision). Lovelace did not provide any articles, guidelines, standards, or even the articles it

supposedly "relied" on to deny the treatment . . . That nurse wrote down the names of three journal articles which he said supported denial (though one was published only in Japanese) . . . It didn't provide the "complete" benefit plan; instead, it provided only two pages from the handbook (the two pages of exclusions!). It had to provide the doctor's recommendation. It didn't. It omitted from the packet the 2-page letter from the doctor who recommended the treatment. It also omitted the actual "request for service" of the BMT from the PCP (which had been dated 4-27-04). Lovelace gave the panel a chronology reporting that the "request" for BMT had been made on May 13, not April 27. (May 13 is within the 5 days of the actual day of denial—May 17—which explains the lie). The panel was chaired by a medical director who indicates that she spent "extra time" on this decision to make sure it was done right. The panel made its decision in less than an hour, start to finish. Yet, this careful doctor admitted she only "scanned" the articles that the world's leading expert in BMT for lupus had personally sent. She ignored calling that expert, who pleaded with Lovelace to call her on the phone before the hearing. The panel denied the treatment because BMT for lupus was in "Phase II clinical trials." Yet, this doctor admits she doesn't even know what is meant by the term "Phase I, II, and III clinical trials."

The next day, Friday, June 18, we received a mailed copy of the internal appeal denial decision.

Robert walked into our bedroom, holding the letter. "There is no way they could have looked at Dr. O'Sullivan's letter yesterday and still mailed this in time for us to get it today. Something's not right."

I was puzzled. "What do you mean?"

"We're denied again." Robert shook his head and walked out with a look of defeat.

In the end, it appeared to us that we lost the appeal based on Lovelace's continued insistence that their Holy Handbook stated that so-called "experimental treatments," such as stem cell transplants, were not covered for lupus patients.

Documents Robert later obtained about the 2-1 decision revealed that the two Lovelace employees voted against us. What a coincidence. Based on all the circumstantial evidence we could muster, the decision to deny my appeal was in before we arrived at the hearing. The panel had no intention of reviewing all the facts, including Dr. O'Sullivan's letter of medical necessity. I believe the vote was taken as soon as we left the building, and a stamp was put on an envelope containing the denial before we left the parking lot. Robert believes that the hearing would have taken place with or without us that day. It's a reasonable assumption based on both past and future actions taken by Lovelace, Ardent, and Cigna employees to provide a prohibitive appeal process.

At the time, we didn't understand why Lovelace had rushed the appeal hearing. I speculated they were empathetic human beings responding to the severity of my condition. Naivety is borne of ignorance, and it leads to more of the same.

Two days after that internal appeal hearing on Saturday, June 19, we received a mailed notice to attend the meeting we had already attended. The postmark was stamped one day after the hearing, and on the same day, we received the denial letter from the internal panel. In other words, we received the internal appeal denial before we received the notice to attend the internal appeal. The bitter reality was that the rush for the hearing had nothing to do with my deteriorating condition. It was a classic case of Lovelace trying to keep from exceeding the State of New Mexico's time limit for the hearing. To add insult to injury, a soon-to-be good friend at the New Mexico Managed Health Care Bureau would reveal a New Mexico statute that should have taken precedence at the hearing. The key phrase is italicized for emphasis:

> You may wish to also review 13.10.17.13; Basis for Initial Certification or Adverse Determination Decisions. When considering whether to certify or deny a health care service requested by a provider or covered person, the health care insurer shall determine whether the requested health care service is covered by the health benefits plan and whether the requested health care service is medically necessary. *A health care insurer shall determine whether the requested health care service is medically necessary even when it determines that a requested health care service is not covered by the health benefits plan.*

On Tuesday, June 22, 2004, Robert took the next step and filed for an external appeal. It seemed clear why Lovelace had not placed the O'Sullivan medical-necessity letter in evidence: It decisively confirmed the "medically necessary" proviso of the State of New Mexico mandate.

Five

External Appeal

On September 9, 2004, Joe Castellano from the Office of Superintendent of Insurance of the New Mexico Public Regulation Commission attended the external appeal hearing. He represented the state in support of us. Joe met us outside the meeting room prior to the session. He was a comforting, father-like figure who did his best to explain the process in which we would be engaged. This was supposed to be a neutral setting, but looking out the window, I could see a huge Lovelace hospital just a hundred yards away. It shared the same parking lot as the building we were in.

Some might call this a meeting of chance, but I like to think it was divine intervention. Robert and I trusted Joe and believed he was a decent human being—but Joe had a past. I confirmed through Justia, a company that makes legal information and resources easy to find online, that in 1995, Joe had been impeached as a New Mexico district judge by the New Mexico Supreme

Court. We decided not to be reproved, and Joe proved honest and up-front about everything we discussed. And unlike many other people who became involved in our case, he did not pry into our personal lives.

The panel was supposed to be composed of two independent physicians and one attorney. We were the first to enter the room. One by one, the panel members entered and took their seats across the table from Robert, Joe, and me. The last person to walk in—it was more of a saunter, as though he was headed to the cafeteria for lunch— was Dr. Harold Sunderman, the medical director for Lovelace. The three-panel members acknowledged him with a nod. Sunderman shook the hand of a man identified as Dr. Bankhurst and sat down.

Before anyone introduced themselves, and before the appeal went on the record, one "nonpartisan" member, Holly R. Harvey, who worked at a law firm representing Lovelace, asked the first question. What Robert and I agreed we heard was, "Do you give up your right to sue us?"

"What?" I asked, dumbfounded. "I just want what my doctor requested—that I receive the stem cell transplant. I do not want to sue anyone." This answer seemed to please her, and she smiled.

Another representative was Arthur Bankhurst, MD, who did contract work for Lovelace. Robert discovered this only because we had been given the wrong packet outlining the hearing, and it contained the contact information and background of every panel member.

After the people around the table introduced themselves, I was invited to present my case. This is from the official transcript of my testimony from that day:

> I have had lupus for the past twelve years ... During the years they have treated me with several medications that Lovelace has provided for me ... Everything that is available to me I have failed to see results or I have rejected the medication ... When I asked at the last hearing if they could give me any alternative besides the stem cell transplant, the room remained silent ... My kidneys have failed. When I'm driving, I forget where I'm going. It's affecting my brain. Can you imagine being with my children, driving somewhere, and not remembering where I am? ... Lovelace has tried everything out there. They have nothing else for me but to deny alternative treatment.

After I finished speaking, the multipronged assault began.

Bankhurst handed out research he had conducted on the National Institutes of Health (NIH) sponsoring stem cell transplants. Then he took the first punch:

> I talked to the National Institutes of Health in Washington, DC. They are recruiting presently for patients with lupus like yourself, and all charges are free. Everything is covered by the government, and they are recruiting right now for just what you are asking. There may even be opportunity to get travel funds, though that can be negotiated. It may not even cost you the price of—

I interrupted. "You know I have five children and do not have money to travel."

Bankhurst pointed his finger at me as he sat up in his seat and continued with a demanding voice:

> Listen to me now. They have travel funds available, and you can request those and you may be able to get those, okay?

Not once did he mention Lovelace's responsibility to provide the transplant or the fact that they had approved it less than twelve hours before it was denied. He insisted that Lovelace had limited resources and that stem cell transplants for lupus are better funded by the government.

"It will all be covered by federal funds and at no expense at all to yourself, co-payment or anything else," Bankhurst said. "I can give you the number to call." In case everybody in the room didn't understand the implications of what he was saying, Bankhurst finished his pitch: "If you don't qualify for this particular study, it's probably unlikely that you would be helped by this kind of treatment anywhere."

The problem was, none of that was true. It's what American media have now come to label "alternative facts." The NIH study was extremely limited, for extremely limited purposes, both for medical and budgetary reasons. Participants in such a study are volunteers who may or may not be compensated at what NIH calls "inconvenience rates," which are determined by the study's principal investigator. The bottom line is that a huge bureaucracy adopts anyone in an NIH study, and that necessarily involves time, scrutiny, and paperwork that involves both the referring physician and the patient.

In case Bankhurst hadn't already done enough damage, the other medical hearing officer, Dr. Seelinger, decided to impeach my Boston doctor. Dr. Traynor had asserted that Medicare reimbursed for this treatment. In a hearing aimed at finding the truth, he would have asked questions like, "Where is the contract that affects this case? Where are the medical records of the patient? Where are the uniform coverage standards?" Instead, Seelinger said the following:

> I just want to make a comment. In the information that was one of the letters from Ann Traynor said that Medicare and Medicaid did cover this, and I called the medical director of Medicare and it is not at this time a covered condition. And I think that's just, as long as we are looking at all the facts, that is a question. They faxed it to me. I have no other questions.

The comments from the panel members appeared to have been rehearsed. How many times had they worked from this script? How many dying people had stood before them as they delivered their lines? If there were such a thing as an empathy meter, would it have flatlined if attached to everyone from Lovelace in that room?

Bankhurst handed me the contact information, phone number, and web address of the National Institutes of Health.

Then the second assault began. Sunderman, the man who had initiated the original denial, broke his silence.

> I think the position of the health plan in this really is not a question of whether this is a treatment for Mrs. Maloney at this point. Clearly, the medical records will show that she has exhausted all other treatments, and this is pretty much what is left to her. Unfortunately, we don't cover experimental investigational procedures.

Before Robert could explode, I stood up.

> What is he saying? Are they going to wait for me to die? When they say they don't accept a phase II clinical trial unless it's an emergency, that is what the handbook says. Why isn't this an emergency? There is nothing else for me. So they will just wait for me to die and expect me to keep paying for insurance until I die.

After the meeting adjourned, I could not stop crying. Robert helped me out of the room with Joe close behind. Looking back, I felt from the moment we walked into the external appeal hearing that it was an ambush to persuade us to seek alternative options to the stem cell transplant. I believed the appeal members had tried to inflict a guilt trip on us for insisting on the transplant.

I could hear the panel members mumbling in the other room, but at that moment, I just wanted to leave.

Joe walked up to us. "I'm so sorry that you had to endure the arrogant indifference of that panel."

"It's my life!" I replied. "Talk about experimenting? Lovelace experimented on me with that IVIG and chemotherapy. Those only have a twenty percent success rate. The stem cell transplant is a phase two clinical trial with an eighty-five percent success rate for curing lupus! If this treatment gives me a healthy five years of life, I'll take them! If I only got one year of healthy life with my children, it'd be worth it. I'm not sure what to call this, but what I am experiencing now isn't life."

Joe called several hours later and said the panel's focus was on alternatives to Lovelace paying $100,000 for the stem cell transplant and not on the underlying medical necessity of the transplant itself and Lovelace's responsibility to provide all necessary care. Joe said he argued on our behalf but that the outcome looked grim. He asked us to try to remain optimistic, and he promised to call as soon as a decision reached his desk. Robert told him he had researched the program Bankhurst recommended and found it was misrepresented at best. Joe asked Robert to write down what he had researched and send a copy to him and his assistant, Tammy Wolf. We did.

> There are a couple of items that came up during our hearing on Thursday, 9/9/04, that I would like to address. The first is the information that was presented by Dr. Bankhurst concerning the National Institutes of Health (NIH)... Dr. Bankhurst made the assumption that this was a viable solution to the problem. He also projected this assumption to

the rest of the panel. He stated that if Zelphoe was not accepted to this program that she would not be accepted by any other one . . . The facts are that the NIH are only looking for 14 people to participate, that the max age is 40, and that gender, age, and medical history will be considered for the participants. They are trying to get a wide spectrum of participants. Even if Zelphoe meets all the eligibility requirements, she could still be rejected, not because she is not eligible but because the NIH has too many qualified females, 39 years old, or persons with certain conditions. We hope this is not the case but it is out of our control.

The other concern is it seemed that Dr. Bankhurst and the medical director for Lovelace, Dr. Sunderman, seem to know each other or seemed to have discussed the matter before the hearing. We are not sure of this, and if we are mistaken, we apologize. But if it is true, we are wondering why Dr. Bankhurst did not recuse himself from the hearing. We appreciate your concern and prompt action to this matter.

* * *

More than two weeks after the external appeal hearing, on September 27, 2004, Robert was picking our daughter Bridgette up from elementary school. As Bridgette got into the car, he answered a call from Joe Castellano. Joe explained that the external appeal panel had upheld the denial but that his office would recommend the superintendent overturn the decision based on the state's statute that says insurance companies operating in New Mexico cover medically necessary procedures. Joe recommended we file an appeal directly to his boss, the superintendent of insurance, while he also filed a request on our behalf in a letter to the superintendent. Joe did so a week later, on October 4.

> [The appeal is denied.] However, Ms. Tammy Wolf and I were of the opinion that such treatment was covered under the plan. The reasoning was set out in a memo submitted to you on September 30, 2004. Enclosed you will find that memo that is the basis for our recommendation and conclusion that it falls under the medical necessity provisos of health plan and mandated pursuant to state insurance regulations, cited herein.
>
> The first treatment requested by the insured and recommended by her treating physician, was initially denied on the basis that it was experimental/investigational, therefore not covered under the plan, subsequently Lovelace reversed itself and approved the new treatment.
>
> After the approved treatment (IVIG) failed, Mrs. Maloney's treating physician requested a new procedure through stem cell transplant being utilized in Boston, Mass. The basis for such request was that the new procedure was a "medical necessity."

Lovelace refused to approve the new "bone marrow treatment" on the grounds that it was experimental/investigational and thus not covered under the plan.

During testimony at the external hearing, it was admitted by Lovelace that they had not offered any "alternative" nor given any other treatment options to her illness, which was determined to be terminal. Their case management personnel had not consulted with the insured or sought other options.

The Boston, Mass. bone marrow treatment program that the insured desired and recommended by her treating physician had been in use for some period and had demonstrated some success. This Lovelace acknowledged as showing "some success," but did not show a high enough amount of trial to be considered a valid non-experimental therapy. Yet when asked what (%) was required to be considered a success or no longer experimental, they could not give an answer.

It was brought out that the new bone marrow treatment program being utilized in Boston was under limited approval of the FDA (which was required before the plan would accept as non-experimental) and results indicated that it had a fairly high success rate for treatment of lupus nephritis.

Furthermore, and most important, under Title 13: Insurance; Chapter 10: Health Insurance; Part 13: Managed Health Care, the following regulation applies: 13.10.17.13 Basis for Initial Certification of Adverse Determination Decisions:

When considering whether to certify or deny a health care service requested by a provider or covered person, the health care insurer shall determine whether the requested health care service is covered by the health benefits plan and whether the requested health care service is medically necessary. A health care insurer shall determine whether the requested health care service is medically necessary even when it determines that a requested health care service is not covered by the health benefits plan, provided that, if a health care insurer denies a requested health care service on the basis of coverage only . . . the superintendent will deem the health care insurer to have conceded that the requested health care service is "MEDICALLY NECESSARY."

Considering all the above, and the fact that the prognosis for the insured (Maloney) indicated that no other treatment was suggested or provided this patient, the end result would be terminal. On this basis it is imperative that the insured receive the treatment prescribed by her treating physician, i.e. bone marrow treatment. It is clear that there is no other alternative, and that this treatment has now entered the realm of "medically necessary" pursuant to the plan and the state insurance regulations, and therefore should be provided to the insured. The health care insurer has conceded that the health care treatment prescribed by the treating physician is now "medically necessary," and thereby legally mandated.

Robert later told me he did his best to explain to Bridgette why some people did not want her mother to get the treatment she needed. When they returned home, Bridgette ran from the car and burst through the front door. "Mom! Mom!" she called out as she bolted into my room, eyes filled with tears, and knelt next to me, wrapping her little arms around my frail neck.

Startled, I asked, "What happened at school, baby? Is everything okay?"

Moments later, Robert walked in and saw us crying in each other's arms. "I'm sorry, hon. I wanted to tell you." He sat on the bed next to us and joined in the hug. The rest of my children came to see why everyone was in tears, and soon, all our children were on the bed, crying, though I don't believe our four-year-old twins fully understood why.

In the days to come, Robert studied how the Public Regulation Commission functioned and what role it played in the healthcare process. His homework proved invaluable later in helping us pinpoint the potential for corruption:

- Five commissioners were elected officials that ran every four years. The commission oversaw industries deemed vital to a citizen's well-being, which included telephone, power, and insurance.

- The superintendent of insurance was appointed by the governor and served at the pleasure of the public regulation commissioners. He was, in effect, the enforcer of the commission with the authority to fine companies that abused public trust or disregarded regulations. At this time, the superintendent was Eric Serna, and the Governor was Bill Richardson.

- The superintendent was also the mediator between insurance companies and the public.

Joe Castellano asked Robert to appeal to Superintendent Eric Serna.

"News travels fast" was my interpretation when my husband explained a telephone conversation he had with Joe Castellano on October 5, 2004, concerning our plea to Serna.

I listened as Robert spoke to Joe on the phone. Robert was expressing his confusion about a recorded message left by Cigna. "You mean the superintendent hasn't made a decision yet? Why did that woman from Cigna lie? Her phone message was specific. She said the superintendent denied the appeal, and now they are closing our file."

Joe assured Robert that was not the case. He insisted that no decision had been made on the part of the superintendent and that our appeal was still on Serna's desk. Joe asked Robert to save the phone message on tape, which had the time and date recorded with it. We did.

Cigna officially closed our case on Friday morning, October 15, 2004, five days before Serna officially denied the request to overturn the external appeal panel's decision on October 20 at 3:59 p.m. The following Wednesday, we received a mailed copy of the superintendent's denial, which was mailed on October 21. The majority of the Final Order from Eric Serna read verbatim from the External Appeals Panel's recommendation:

> On September 24, 2004, the External Review Panel submitted to the Superintendent the following unanimous findings:
>
> The Lovelace Health Plan 2004 Member Handbook clearly excludes procedures which the Plan's Medical Director determines are experimental or investigational;
>
> The stem cell transplant Mrs. Maloney is requesting for treatment of her lupus nephritis is experimental at this time;
>
> The requested stem cell transplant is, therefore, not a covered benefit under the member's plan.
>
> Based upon the entire record in this matter and the above-stated recommendation decision by the

External Review Panel, the Superintendent hereby finds the External Review Panel's recommended decision to be well taken and should be adopted.

IT IS THEREFORE ORDERED that the attached September 24, 2004, recommended decision by the External Review Panel is ADOPTED.

DONE AND ORDERED on this the 20th day of October 2004.

We received official notification from the superintendent twelve days after Cigna closed our file based on the superintendent's decision. Cigna closed our file five days *before* the superintendent even made his decision.

We immediately called Joe when we received the letter. He confirmed the decision.

From my perspective, the Review Panel had ignored the law and issued me a death sentence. I had to come to grips with the reality that my days were numbered, and I had better make the most of the time I had left. I drew close to my family, and they drew close to me.

Was this what acceptance—the final stage of grief—felt like?

Six

Unwelcome

Robert held strong in his confidence in the system. He planned to go to Santa Fe and expose Serna's blatant disregard of the law to the Public Regulation Commissioners. Robert was certain they would overturn the denial and possibly dismiss Serna.

Someone in Santa Fe should have sent us a note saying, "Welcome to state politics! By the way, you aren't welcome here!"

On Thursday, October 28, 2004, we dressed in our Sunday best and drove sixty miles to the PRC building in the state capital. Robert made five cassette copies of the phone message from Cigna, five copies of the signed, dated, and time-stamped decision from Serna, a brief explanation of the relevance of each, and a letter for consideration. He sealed them in five manila envelopes addressed to each commissioner. This is what Robert wrote.

New Mexico Public Regulation Commissioners:

We appreciate your attention to the matter of Lovelace Health Plan's denial of treatment for Zelphoe Maloney. We feel that Zelphoe's condition is extremely urgent and needs immediate action. Lovelace's denial of medical services has generated great mental anguish for us, and in the case of Zelphoe, great physical distress. We obtained our insurance in good faith and expected Lovelace to provide for our medical needs.

Let us look at the handbook at what Lovelace told us to expect from them. They say that we "will be treated with dignity as a person and receive assistance in a prompt, courteous manner" (HB, p. 5). "This pertaining from any appropriate or medically necessary treatment you receive. This right exists regardless of cost of benefit coverage. This is required unless there is an emergency and your life and health are in serious danger." (HB, p. 5) We feel that Zelphoe's life is in danger, as does her treating physician, Dr. O'Sullivan. Lovelace also states we should follow our physician's advice and consider the likely results if we do not (HB, p. 6).

After talking with Dr. O'Sullivan, we found that a stem cell transplant was our only choice. According to the handbook, the plan covers human organ transplants, including bone marrow (HB, p. 18). Lovelace states that its denial was determined on the basis that stem cell transplants for lupus patients are not covered and that the medical director determined that the treatment was not necessary. Lovelace, in its own words, admits that the handbook is open for interpretation. "The role of the Internal Medical Review is to interpret benefits as outlined in the Member's Handbook and Certificate" (Exhibit C, p. 24). As we have seen in a previous interpretation from Lovelace, "Intravenous Immunoglobulin may be covered in the management of members when medical necessity has been established" (Exhibit K, p. 130). As Dr. O'Sullivan states in his recommendation letter, "Autologous stem cell transplantation offers the only possible hope," which exemplifies Zelphoe's medical necessity. Even though Lovelace determined that immunoglobulin is experimental and expensive, they chose to let Zelphoe take the treatment (Exhibit H, p. 94). We only ask that you do not let the interpretation of a few people with strong ties to Lovelace deny a loving mother of five her medically necessary treatment. We hope that your interpretation of the evidence will allow her a chance at life.

We had met several PRC candidates while they were campaigning, but we had never tried to work with them. As we walked up to the PRC building, Robert anticipated what the outcome would be, but I was intimidated by the mere thought of challenging the superintendent.

At first, we were met with big smiles and friendly handshakes, but the more envelopes we handed out and the more commissioners we met, the colder the welcome became. E. Shirley Baca was one of the first commissioners we met. She was a petite, well-dressed woman who carried herself with a no-nonsense attitude. She seemed genuinely concerned and spoke to us as peers, not in a condescending fashion. Some of the commissioners were not in, so we dropped envelopes off for them. Before we could reach Commissioner Ben Ray Lujan Jr.'s office to leave the last envelope, an older man in a good suit approached us and asked about our business. Robert took this opportunity to express his frustration with Eric Serna. The man offered to take the last envelope for Commissioner Lujan, but Robert politely declined and continued to Lujan's office. Later, we discovered that the older man was Eric Serna's right-hand man, Joe Ruiz, deputy superintendent of insurance.

Once Lujan's secretary introduced us and we explained why we had come to see him, Robert handed the last envelope to Ben. "Here is the evidence."

"I'm sorry, Mr. Maloney, but I'm not sure if I should take this from you since it's about an open case before the superintendent."

"What do you mean? He serves at your pleasure," Robert fired back.

"What I mean is we need to follow procedure. As it stands right now, I have no jurisdiction over the superintendent's findings."

"But you can fire him for just cause," I interjected.

"Let's not rush into things. It takes a majority of the commissioners to vote for dismissal. Let's see how this plays out."

"We don't have time to let things play out," Robert insisted. "My wife only has a few months to live if she doesn't get the stem cell transplant."

"I assure you, Mr. Maloney, we have to let all legal avenues be explored before the commission can consider looking into this matter. Even then, we may have no legal grounds to intervene." Ben handed the envelope back to Robert. "I wish there were something I could do. But be assured I will follow this as it progresses."

Robert's enthusiasm evaporated, and although it didn't seem possible, I felt even more helpless than before we entered the building. It seemed to both of us that no one who was in a position to help cared that I was living on borrowed time.

Robert stood motionless in front of Ben Lujan Jr. Robert later told me that at that moment, the reality of political intervention replaced his perception of public service.

I grabbed Robert's arm and urged him to leave. On the way out, Robert picked up all the envelopes we had dropped off at the other commissioners' offices without question or resistance from anyone. I felt they were glad we had picked them up—perhaps someone had told them not to look at the information—but I couldn't be sure. As we entered the elevator, we noticed Joe Ruiz peeking around a corner, watching us and smiling. In our haste to leave, we had forgotten to stop by Joe Castellano's office.

The next day, Joe Castellano called us to explain how our visit had started whispers and rumors inside the PRC and especially in the Office of the Superintendent of Insurance. Joe also asked us to call our commissioner, Herb H. Hughes, to discuss possible options.

    Robert phoned Hughes at home. The call obviously annoyed him. After Robert briefly explained our circumstances, Hughes replied, "I'm leaving office in a couple of months. I don't want to stir the pot. You'll have to wait for Jason Marks to be sworn in." Then he hung up.

Seven

A Shot in the Dark

Joe Castellano relayed a message from Eric Serna asking us to sign a request Serna had him produce. The request was for another appeal to the superintendent's office for consideration.

> Dear Mr. Serna:
>
> My wife (Zelphoe) and I would respectfully request that you reconsider your order dated October 20, 2004, regarding the external review involving my wife's treatment issues with Lovelace. We ask you to grant us a re-hearing before the External Review Panel, which met on September 9, 2004. New information has surfaced which the panel did not consider or have an opportunity to review. It is our belief, if this new evidence is presented, that the

panel will ultimately reach a new recommendation and a different conclusion from that reported by them on September 24, 2004.

Therefore, please allow us our request for this new hearing. My wife, my children, and I thank you for any efforts you make on our behalf.

There were big problems with this request. First, neither Robert nor I write in this style. Second, it was backdated to October 27, 2004. Third, we had no new evidence.

Robert and I weren't sure what to do. Joe called Robert several more times during the next few days. Robert felt Joe was trying to tell him something indirectly, but we were not sure what that might be. I found Robert's handwritten notes on why we shouldn't sign the request:

Reasons not to request another panel hearing:

1. Gives Lovelace the opportunity to question medical necessity.
2. According to Reg. 13.10.17.13 the superintendent has the authority to overturn the panel; he does not need another panel review.
3. It will take more time.
4. It allows the superintendent a way out to clean his hands.
5. We need a lawyer.

Our initial attempts to secure legal counsel yielded nothing. We spoke to a dozen attorneys; they shut down when we mentioned Eric Serna. The sole attorney willing to take our case, a young man in his twenties, wanted $20,000 in cash up front as a retainer. "You'll need to cover monthly expenses," he added. "I can't afford to be out-of-pocket on something like this." We didn't have the money.

That evening, after the children went to bed, Robert left for his office. The house was silent as I lay in bed, reasoning that all this must have a purpose. I turned on the television and suddenly remembered a program I had watched years earlier. I couldn't remember the name of the movie, the name of the woman whose life it was based on, or the actress who starred in it—only that it was about insurance corruption and abuse. I called Robert at his office and asked him to search the web. After a tense moment, he found a list of all the Lifetime for Women movies and started reading them to me in alphabetical order. When he mentioned *Damaged Care*, I yelled, "That's it! It's about Linda Peeno, a doctor who fights against insurance company abuse. Laura Dern plays the doctor who risks everything to become a whistleblower and advocate."

Robert asked me to wait on the phone while he searched for more information. "Linda Peeno has her website," he told me, "but don't get your hopes up. It's five years old, and I'm not sure if it's still active."

"Just try!" I insisted.

Robert asked me to wait while he read Linda Peeno's testimony before Congress:

I wish to begin by making a public confession: in the spring of 1987, as a physician, I caused the death of a man. No person or group has held me accountable for this—for this was half a million dollar savings to my employer. In fact, this act secured my reputation as a "good" company doctor and ensured my advancement in the health care industry. In little more than a year, I went from making a few hundred dollars per week to an annual six-figure income.

In all my work, I had one primary duty: to use my medical expertise for the financial benefit of the organization. According to the managed care industry, it is not an ethical issue to sacrifice a human being for a "savings." I was repeatedly told that I was not denying care. I was only denying payment.

I am not an ethicist whose opinions have come from a few books. For me, the ethical issues were born in the trenches, fed by the pain I know I caused. If I am an expert, it is in how managed care maims and kills patients.

I am here today to tell you about the dirty work of managed care.

"She seems like the person we need to help us," Robert said. "She lives in Kentucky. There's an e-mail address for her at the bottom of the web page. I'll send her a message."

Dr. Peeno, my wife has lupus. She has been fighting it for twelve years. She has exhausted all medical and nonmedical treatments except a stem cell transplant. Dr. Frank O'Sullivan, her specialist for the past four years, told us a stem cell transplant is her only hope. He referred her to Dr. Ann Traynor for the procedure. Our HMO denied her claim on the basis that it is experimental. We have appealed their decision three times. The last time, the superintendent of insurance of New Mexico upheld the denial. We discovered that there's a state regulation in New Mexico that mandates that the superintendent overrule the decision in the case of medical necessity. We do not understand why the HMO would feel comfortable enough to close our case a week before they received official notice. We can fax you all the information if you wish. An insider told us that we did not have a chance from the beginning. We suspected as much, given the circumstances of the denial by the superintendent. Please, if you can help, call, fax, or e-mail us at . . .

That night, for the first time in a long time, I felt a little peace.

In the morning, Robert's phone rang, waking us up. You could have blown him over with a breath as he stood, looking at me in disbelief. I wanted to jump, although that was physically impossible for me to do when I heard him say, "Yes, Mrs. Peeno, she's here." Robert handed me the phone.

Feeling more hopeful than I had since I'd first heard about the stem cell option, I anxiously told her that the superintendent was trying to force us to sign something he wrote to request another panel hearing. Linda was confident she could help and seemed to have answers to all my questions or at least an understanding of what we were going through. I listened closely as she advised us not to request another appeal or sign anything from the superintendent or Lovelace. She asked me to wait for her to contact some attorneys in Las Cruces on our behalf. If that didn't work, she knew some attorneys in Pennsylvania who loved taking cases that revolved around questionable insurance company policies.

    I was amazed at Linda's knowledge of insurance tactics and the lengths insurance executives would go to save money. By the end of the conversation, I felt like a fighter again.

Eight

Maloneys vs. Goliaths

Within an hour of speaking with Linda, we received a call from attorney Bill Webber. Although we were doubtful they would take our case, we accepted the invitation to meet with Bill Webber, Bob Mayfield, and Joel Newton 220 miles south of Albuquerque in Las Cruces, a midsized city in southern New Mexico, on November 4, 2004.

The law office of Mayfield, Webber & Newton was operated out of a converted Circle K convenience store. Still, it was lavishly decorated, with leather couches, Southwestern-style furnishings, and a large, round mahogany table in the conference room. Robert and I entered the office, where we met Bill, a tall, slender, hippie-cowboy type in his fifties from Texas; Joel Newton, a conservatively dressed athletic fellow in his thirties; and Bob Mayfield, a lanky cowboy lawyer in his late seventies. It was apparent that Joel and Bill were surprised by my 90-pound appearance, and Bob was visibly upset by my frail condition. I moved like a woman three times my age, and Robert had to help me with each step.

"My God!" Bob exclaimed. "How in the world did your doctor let your health deteriorate to this level? Come and sit down."

"Bob," Joel interjected, "I'm going to call and see if we can get the studio. We need to get anything she wants to tell us video-recorded today."

Bob and Bill nodded in agreement. Joel stepped out of the office, and the four of us took seats around the conference table. It didn't dawn on me until years later that the lawyers wanted a video because they felt I might not live much longer.

As Robert and I described our experience for the video file, Joel was mesmerized. Bill and Bob looked as though they were hearing an old, familiar story.

In the end, I believe five key factors converged that day that started all five of us on a trek that would forever change our lives. First, Bill Webber had a compassionate soul and a commitment to protecting the little person. Second, the opportunity for Bill to work with an advocate such as Linda Peeno nudged him in favor of taking our case. Third, Joel Newton was a devout member of the traditional Church of Christ. I saw in his eyes that his attitude was shifting in our favor when Robert mentioned we shared the same faith. Fourth, Bob had attended the New Mexico Military Institute, the same one my husband graduated from as a young man. Bob was hard to read and a veteran of the political system in Santa Fe, having once run for governor. His years of life experience allowed him to hide his emotions well. But when I mentioned the Institute, Bob's smile left me no doubt that he was on board.

The final convincing factor was my condition. Compassion filled the faces of these three men as we discussed the injustice that had left me virtually one breath from death. Everyone in the room began to cry as I expressed how I felt about myself: "I'm not a mother or a wife, and I'm not even sure I'm a human being."

After the interview, we sat down to talk about the next steps. Bob Mayfield spoke first. "We'll have to discuss it among ourselves before we decide on accepting your case."

"Any help would be greatly appreciated," I replied. "As of now, we have nothing."

"We'll get back to you tomorrow," Bill said.

Joel didn't say a word, but I could tell by the look in his eyes that he was ready for a fight. And by this time, so was I.

* * *

The morning after our first meeting with the attorneys, my husband received a call from Bill Webber. Robert came into the bedroom and announced, "They took our case." I noticed something I hadn't seen in a long time: hope in his eyes.

It was fortunate that we hadn't requested another appeal to Eric Serna. Bill told us that doing so would have negated the first appeal and possibly eliminated our ability to sue Lovelace and the Office of the Superintendent of Insurance. In a future conversation with Joe Castellano, he gave us the ugly background on the second appeal letter. He knew the idea was flawed but believed that someone else in the office was eavesdropping. Joe confided to Robert, and later to Joel, that Eric Serna had promised him a promotion if he could persuade us to sign the new request. Luckily,

Robert had picked up on Joe's halfhearted attempt and put off the decision until we spoke to Bill Webber, even though Robert and I trusted Joe.

In the end, Joe Castellano became a good friend. Don't get me wrong—we were repeatedly told about the scandals he'd been involved in while he was a district judge, but in our minds, Joe's scandals were overtaken by his kindnesses. Right after Serna denied our appeal, Joe urged Robert to attend a private Con Alma Health Foundation annual banquet that night and take note of the attendees. Con Alma is a Santa Fe-based organization that describes its mission as seeking "to improve the health status and access to health care services, and advocates for a health policy, which will address the unmet needs of all New Mexicans." Joe's phone call about the event was probably the single most important call of our entire ordeal. It shed a bright light on what we were facing.

In late November 2004, Robert sneaked into the Con Alma banquet, an invitation-only black-tie event. When he arrived in his best suit, he felt completely underdressed. At the entrance was a check-in table where staff members were verifying invitations. Robert stood around, watching for an opportunity to sneak past them. He noticed several high-profile politicians in the lobby. One was former New Mexico governor Bruce King, a slim man in his eighties with pure white hair, who was slightly hunched and walked with a cane. Robert had only met him once at a fundraiser. As King approached, Robert walked up and gave him a big hug. "Governor King! Good to see you!"

Robert kept his arm around the former governor as if they were old friends. One of the staff members checked the invitation and handed King a seating chart, saying, "Glad you could attend, Governor."

Robert ignored the man checking invitations and kept in conversation with King as they walked into the banquet. Then Robert politely excused himself and continued inside the 14,000-square-foot ballroom. As he slowly ventured farther in, he noticed large round tables covered with silken tablecloths and adorned with champagne bottles, roses, and brass plaques bearing the names of different insurance companies, including Lovelace. He estimated that there were at least fifty tables that could hold up to twenty people each. The room was almost filled as guests mingled and indulged in free drinks and hors d'oeuvres. In an attempt to blend in, Robert asked for a drink.

After Robert took a sip, he looked up. The ceiling was decorated with large, square tray panels outlined by crown molding, with a chandelier in each square. Blue and purple lights reflected from the ceiling and sparkled on the tables below. At the far end of the room hung two large projection screens. The words *Con Alma* were emblazoned above the image of a crying child in a hospital bed. Under the image were the words *We Care*.

Robert considered this spectacle for a moment: *Why are the insurance companies that the superintendent of insurance regulates buying tables at a fundraiser hosted by the superintendent of insurance?*

Robert turned and found Eric Serna standing in front of him, dressed in a designer suit and Corfam wingtips.

Serna gave him a suspicious look. "Have we met?"

Robert extended his hand, saying, "Yes, but it's been a while."

"I can't quite recall," Serna said as he shook Robert's hand.

Robert smiled. "It was at the Roundhouse. How is everything

at the PRC?" The Roundhouse is the nickname for New Mexico's state capitol building, considered by some to be the most unique capitol building in the country.

"The Roundhouse?"

Robert let go of Serna's hand. "You'll have to excuse me. I must find my wife."

Serna smiled. "Of course."

Robert walked away and breathed a sigh of relief. A few moments later, he heard Serna announce over the intercom, "The Con Alma presentation is about to begin. Please find your way to your seats."

The attendees lingering in the outside corridor headed into the banquet hall. The staff who had checked people in started to clean off the check-in tables. Robert noticed one lady tossing a stack of booklets into the trash. He walked over, and when no one was watching, he reached into the trash can and pulled out a booklet.

One staff member asked, "Can I help you?"

Robert calmly turned toward the man and said, "Mr. Serna asked me to save one of these for him."

"Will one be enough?"

Robert smiled. "This will be fine. Thank you."

The man nodded and continued with the cleanup. Robert thumbed through the booklet for a couple of seconds and then rushed out to his car.

Robert was certain he had uncovered evidence that could help with our case. But he didn't realize that the list of insurance companies who had bought tickets from the superintendent of insurance would not be as important as who gave out the tickets and who accepted them.

The list of companies who had bought tickets included the following, in alphabetical order: Aflac, American General, American Physicians Assurance Inc., Blue Cross Blue Shield of New Mexico, Daniels Insurance, Delta Dental of New Mexico, Fairfax, Globe Life Insurance, Heartland Alliance, Independent Insurance Agents of New Mexico, Lovelace Sandia Health Systems, Loya Insurance Company, Molina Healthcare Inc., Mora Community Health Service, Mountain States Insurance Group, New Mexico Mutual Group, Presbyterian Healthcare Services, Santa Fe Auto Insurance Company, State Farm Insurance, Talbot Insurance, Title Insurance Industry of New Mexico, University of New Mexico Hospital, and Wachovia.

According to the best information we had, the list of attendees who received tickets but did not pay for them included the following:

- Governor Bill Richardson's wife, Barbara Richardson
- Lieutenant Governor Diane Denish
- Former governor Bruce King
- New Mexico Supreme Court justices Patricio Serna and Edward L. Chavez
- Future New Mexico Supreme Court justice Barbara Vigil
- Court of Appeals judge James Wechsler
- Superintendent of Insurance Eric Serna and his wife, Barbara
- Deputy Superintendent of Insurance Joe Ruiz

- President pro tem of the New Mexico Senate, Manny Aragon
- State senators Richard Martinez and Cynthia Nava
- State representative Jim Trujillo
- New Mexico Attorney General Patricia Madrid
- PRC commissioners David King and Linda Lovejoy
- PRC commissioners elect Ben Ray Lujan Jr. and Jason Marks

The Con Alma banquet was attended by the Who's Who of prominent New Mexicans, paid for by the Who's Who of the insurance industry, and hosted by the superintendent of insurance. At least Robert got a drink out of it.

Eric Serna orchestrated the restructuring of Blue Cross Blue Shield when they wanted to go from not-for-profit to for-profit in 2001. The restructure created Con Alma, whose mission was to provide health care to children in New Mexico. Although it had assets close to $30 million at that time, Robert and I could only find where it funded thousands of dollars for children. News reports revealed that someone used a large part of the money to buy and renovate prime office space in downtown Santa Fe for employees and board members, including then-Con Alma president Eric Serna. The story "Nonprofit's Home: $800,000," written by investigative journalist Mike Gallagher, was published in the *Albuquerque Journal* on Sunday, May 9, 2004. Here is an excerpt:

> A nonprofit foundation set up to help provide health care to poor people and medically underserved communities is spending $800,000 to buy and renovate a Santa Fe home for its headquarters.

The split vote by the board of the Con Alma Foundation did not sit well with some members.

Board member Barbara McAneny said she voted against the purchase.

"We have a part-time staff, a phone and a fax machine," said McAneny, an Albuquerque physician. "What do we need with an $800,000 headquarters?"

...

The foundation, founded in 2001 with proceeds from the sale of the nonprofit Blue Cross Blue Shield insurance company, has assets of more than $26 million. The foundation approved $700,000 in grants to be distributed this year and expects to distribute a minimum of $1 million next year.

Eric Serna, chairman of the Con Alma board and the state insurance commissioner, defended the purchase as financially sound.

...

McAneny said she believes the foundation could have found others to donate office space or it could have been purchased for less somewhere else.

Con Alma was formed in 2001 with $15 million when the nonprofit Blue Cross and Blue Shield health insurer was sold to a for-profit company, Health Care Services Corp., which also agreed to pay $5 million to Con Alma over five years.

In 2003, the foundation received another $3.5 million from a settlement over the sale of Los Alamos Medical Center to Province HealthCare . . .

Serna ordered the creation of Con Alma in approving the sale and settlement supervised by Attorney General Patricia Madrid.

The Con Alma banquet was a glittery mask for a deformed face. Serna was responsible for regulating and enforcing regulations on insurance companies in New Mexico. Yet Serna and his subordinates contacted insurance companies to solicit contributions for Con Alma. Joe Castellano, an insider at the PRC, confided to us that Serna insisted Lovelace and other insurance companies buy tables for the banquet and recommended how many seats they should buy. In fact, Lovelace was asked to buy thousands of dollars of tickets just days before Serna upheld the external appeal that condemned me to a death sentence. This might partially explain why Cigna closed my file days before Serna made his final decision on my case. I later discovered this in a letter addressed to Bill Madison, which Joel Newton gave to Robert. Madison would play a key role in our case in the future.

Zelphoe found out about the denial because Cigna called and left a recorded voice mail message . . . The problem was that the superintendent hadn't gotten the file yet, hadn't read the appeal, and hadn't "officially" ruled. But, dutifully, he did rule in favor of Lovelace two days later. That was a few weeks after the $50,000 donation from Lovelace to Con Alma, and about the same time as the mega-banquet sponsored by Lovelace, at whose table President Serna sat, along with multiple dignitaries, very near three Supreme Court justices. Con Alma was the superintendent's "favorite charity," his self-described "baby," and the only charity advertised on the Superintendent of Insurance's official state website.

Serna handed out tickets bought by insurance companies at his pleasure to prominent New Mexico political figures. Any reasonable person would conclude that this represents a conflict of interest.

As president of Con Alma, Serna annually received tens of thousands of dollars in perks, including travel, meals, and office space. According to an *Albuquerque Journal* investigative article published June 30, 2006:

> Con Alma Health Foundation, a nonprofit set up to improve the health of underserved New Mexicans, spent more than $50,000 last year on travel, meals and entertainment.

From 2002 through the end of 2005, Con Alma's tab totaled more than $142,000 in those expense categories, according to IRS filings.

With then-state Insurance Superintendent Eric Serna serving as Con Alma board president, the foundation during those years received more than $200,000 from companies he regulated. Another $146,000 in donations came from banks that did work for his insurance division.

Con Alma's board of trustees asked him in May for the credit card reimbursement because Serna had no supporting documentation for the charges.

They included $442 at the Hotel Del Coronado near San Diego; $1,006 at the Surf & Sand Hotel in Laguna Beach, Calif.; $528 at the Waldorf Astoria in New York and $482 at the Market Inn Restaurant in Washington, D.C.

Con Alma officials have said that they didn't know whether the charges were improper but that Serna's repayment rendered the question moot. The undocumented charges spanned from 2002 to early 2006.

Perhaps most politicians did not know who bought their tickets for the banquet. Perhaps they thought Serna was just being a nice guy.

Nine

The Lone Media Voice

The abuse of power Eric Serna displayed in his handling of Con Alma fundraising caught the eye of a single journalist, Mike Gallagher. The morning after the banquet, Robert called Joel Newton and told him about the event. Joel seemed unimpressed but asked Robert to send him the seating booklet he had recovered. It was apparent in a phone conversation I had with my attorneys that upon review of the booklet, Bill, Joel, and Bob were astonished. The booklet linked prominent New Mexico government officials to a pay-to-play scandal headed by the New Mexico superintendent of insurance. And to complicate matters, Serna was a good friend of Governor Bill Richardson.

    Richardson was a relative nobody when he decided to enter the political arena. His first target was congressman for the third congressional seat in New Mexico. Richardson solicited the help of longtime northern New Mexico political advocate Eric Serna, who cemented Richardson's victory as third district representative. The two would become almost inseparable from then on. Mike Gallagher went relentlessly after scandals involving Bill Richardson or Eric Serna, and there were many he covered in the *Albuquerque Journal*. In an article published on Friday, May 19, 2006, he and Colleen Heild outlined Serna's troubling past. They cited many times in Serna's 29 years of government experience that he strayed from ethical practices, as well as legal ones. But the most glaring offense was his relationship with Con Alma Health Care Foundation.

Ten days before our story broke in the newspaper on a Sunday morning, January 23, 2005, we experienced several strange occurrences. Every morning, when Robert left to take the children to school, he noticed a seemingly unattended late-model white van parked across the street from our home. After a week, he finally asked our neighbors if it belonged to them or if they were getting work done on their home. No one knew anything about the van. In normal circumstances, I guess I should have been frightened, but actually, I didn't care about the strange van. Now I see this cruel tactic for what it was: an attempt to follow and intimidate a person who was fighting for her life. The Sunday our story broke was the last time we saw the van. In addition, when we used our cell phones, we heard unexplained background noise and occasional clicking sounds. A friend in the communication industry told me that what I described is common when a third party monitors a phone.

On Saturday night, before the story broke, Robert took me out for dinner. After we were seated, another couple entered the restaurant and asked for the table next to us. Robert and I were discussing the upcoming article, and the man sitting next to us kept leaning in to listen.

Robert felt uncomfortable and stood up. "Do you need something?" he asked.

The man and woman also stood up. The man clicked something on his belt and said, "We were just leaving." The pair quickly left the restaurant.

I didn't understand Robert's actions until he explained that he had noticed the same man at our salon, bank, and Bridgett's school on several occasions over the past two weeks. Someone had us under surveillance, but we still don't know if it was Lovelace or Eric Serna.

Robert and I were not certain when the story would run. As usual, on Sunday morning Robert drove to the corner gas station to get a coffee and a paper. Robert greeted the clerk as he walked in and headed for the coffee. As he filled his cup, Robert asked, "Anything interesting in the paper?"

The clerk picked up a bundle of newspapers from the floor and placed them on the rack. "Hold on, I'll open a bundle up," he said. Robert walked to the counter as the clerk cut the strap and picked up a copy. "Just some woman holding a child." The clerk showed Robert the cover.

Robert dropped his coffee on the floor and reached for the paper. "That's my wife and daughter!" he exclaimed.

The clerk leaned across the counter and grabbed a handful of rags.

After a breathless moment, Robert said, "I'm sorry, let me get that."

Back in the car, Robert sat down and began to read the front page. Halfway through, he looked up to heaven through the windshield and said, "Thank you, God! We have a chance." He began to cry.

It was the controversy of the seating booklet Robert had retrieved at the Con Alma banquet that had landed a picture of me with our four-year-old daughter Hermione on the front page of the *Albuquerque Journal* in a story by Mike Gallagher titled "Under Fire."

> Eric Serna is the state superintendent of insurance. He is also head of the Con Alma Foundation, which has received more than $100,000 in contributions from the industry Serna regulates.
>
> This dual role is under fire, sparked by a recent case in which he upheld an HMO's decision refusing a bone marrow transplant for a woman with lupus.
>
> "It is the clearest case of conflict of interest I have ever seen," said Sen. Mary Kay Papen, D-Las Cruces. "We have to do something."
>
> It's more than a question of ethics for Zelphoe Maloney. It's a question of life and death. . . .
>
> "I want to be here to see my children grow," Maloney said. "I've missed too much time with them because of this (lupus)."

A panel appointed by Serna upheld the denial, and Serna affirmed that ruling.

"I found nothing that would have allowed me to rule in the Maloneys' favor," he said in a Journal interview.

Lovelace Sandia declined to comment on the case because it is in litigation.

The case has been a catalyst for action on several fronts.

At Papen's urging, the Legislative Finance Committee has ordered a review of how the Insurance Division[1] has handled consumer complaints.

The Public Regulation Commission agreed last week to ask the Legislature to change state law so the commission could hear appeals of Serna's decisions.

The PRC is reviewing a reorganization of the Insurance Division and trying to decide whether it can legally move consumer insurance complaints and appeals of HMO decisions out of Serna's division . . .

Zelphoe Maloney and her husband, Robert . . . contend in their appeal to district court that Serna was

---

[1] The Insurance Division was later renamed the Office of Superintendent of Insurance.

biased because Lovelace Sandia is a contributor to the nonprofit health-care foundation Serna heads. It is an issue that has raised concern with some in state government...

Serna, in an interview, denied any conflict of interest and says he doesn't actively solicit donations on behalf of the Con Alma Healthcare Foundation.

"I don't have to," Serna said, "to criticize me is wrong. I've given my heart and soul to this organization and I'm proud of the work it has done."

Later he said, "I promote Con Alma, damn right. I promote its mission. I do not ask people to contribute."

But others are concerned about Serna's dual role.

"Overall Eric (Serna) has done a good job, but this is a real problem," Public Regulation Commissioner David King said in an interview. "He has a real problem wearing two hats in these cases."

Serna said he has ruled in favor of patients on other occasions. "But the external review panel found nothing to allow me to rule in favor of the Maloneys," he said.

The PRC discussed the issue last week.

While the numbers are in dispute, preliminary research by commissioners indicated there are 400 to 500 consumer insurance complaints each year. Between 35 and 40 reach the external review panel.

Commissioners say it appears 80 to 90 percent of the rulings in recent years have favored insurance companies . . .

The Maloneys said they initially thought their appeal to the state Insurance Division had gone well.

"We were naive," Robert Maloney said. "When we kept losing the internal appeals, I kept telling Zelphoe that we would get a fair shake from the State . . . "

The Maloneys said that on Sept. 28 they received a call from a Lovelace official telling them Serna had denied their appeal . . . "That's when we knew something was wrong," Robert Maloney said.

Eric Serna considers the Con Alma Healthcare Foundation "like one of my children" and resents an implication that his dual role constitutes a conflict of interest . . . The foundation's annual

$100-a-plate banquet is well supported by the insurance industry...

Legal considerations are one thing. Political considerations involved in taking on Serna are another. He is a longtime fundraiser for the Democratic Party, and he has a close relationship with Gov. Bill Richardson dating back to Richardson's election to Congress.

His political stature was evident last week during Richardson's state-of-the-state speech. Serna was sitting in the guest section with the state Supreme Court, Sen. Jeff Bingaman, and Rep. Tom Udall. Public Regulation commissioners were off to the side in a far less prominent location.

But newly elected chairman Ben R. Lujan apparently is willing to take some risks. "To do our job protecting consumers will take some changes," Lujan said. "We have to take a proactive role in legislative changes." Lujan and three other commissioners decided they would seek legislation allowing consumers to appeal decisions from the Insurance Division to the commission.

Serna pointed out that consumers already have a right of appeal to state court.

Lujan said that can be far more expensive than an administrative appeal to the commission... A group of Las Cruces attorneys led by former Democratic state Rep. Bobby Mayfield have been representing the Maloneys pro bono.

"I've never seen a conflict of interest like this," Mayfield said. "When people get the type of power Mr. Serna has, they get reckless... In a lot of cases, issues like conflict of interest or due process are just abstract issues," Mayfield said. "But in this case, they are having a real impact on people's lives."

The Maloneys haven't given up on a transplant for Zelphoe, regardless of how their legal battle is resolved.

The family, already strapped by medical expenses, has decided to try to raise money to have the bone marrow procedure done at Northwestern University. The cost is estimated at between $50,000 and $100,000.

In a conversation years after the ordeal, Joel Newton best described Mike Gallagher's role: "The power of the press! Mike Gallagher getting Zelphoe's picture on the front page of the *Albuquerque Journal* and telling her story .. forced enough of the New Mexico corruption out into the public and started making the politicians concerned they were no longer going to be able to bury her .. because somebody in the press was paying attention."

Ten

A Powerful Ally

E. Shirley Baca was elected to safeguard the citizens of New Mexico from greedy corporate interests, and she displayed the integrity to act on her promise. But she was just one commissioner against the corrupt political machine in her political party. We asked for help from representatives from both major political parties, but all seemed afraid of the "Democrat Machine" in New Mexico.

After Eric Serna had asked Joe Castellano to persuade Robert and me to request a second appeal and the Con Alma scandal hit the press, Shirley asked Joe to help her set up a meeting with Robert and me at her PRC office. We were leery. So far, we have heard a lot of rhetoric from PRC commissioners King and Lujan in person and in their press statements about how they were prohibited by law from helping. Jason Marks, the PRC commissioner for the district where Robert and I lived, also gave his opinion in a letter. Marks forwarded a copy to us on February 5, 2005.

Dear Eric:

As I have expressed to you previously, I am concerned about conflict of interest posed by your concurrent service as insurance superintendent and as president of the Con Alma Foundation. It is my desire that we resolve those conflicts in a manner that best serves the public interest, and to that end, I will be asking that the commission make this a discussion topic for the February 10, 2005, public work session...

The work of Con Alma contributes to our state's future, and I commend you for your very deep personal commitment to those efforts. Given the congruence between Con Alma's mission and the public interest, I don't perceive an inherent conflict between your leadership role at Con Alma and your holding the office of insurance superintendent.

However, two aspects of your (and Con Alma's) activities must be addressed. The most important of these arises from Con Alma's fundraising amongst insurance companies, trade associations, and others who have an interest in your decisions as insurance superintendent. Regardless of whether contributions are being solicited from regulated entities or merely being accepted, I believe that these contributions pose a real conflict of interest, not just an "appearance" of a conflict. While some have emphasized how conflicts can arise in your review of appeals under the Managed Care Act, the conflicts are far broader, potentially affecting all areas of insurance regulation; e.g., title insurance rate setting, agent and company licensing, etc.

The second area that gives rise to concern is the potential for time spent on foundation business to interfere with the discharge of your duties as superintendent. While I am not aware of any specific incidents or problems in this area, the public is entitled to assurance that tax dollars, in the form of your salary, are not unduly subsidizing Con Alma.

Obviously, both of the above concerns would be satisfied by your resignation from the Con Alma Foundation...

Please be prepared to address these matters at the February 10 work session.

Upon Joe's insistence, we agreed to meet with Shirley Baca an hour before the February 17 PRC meeting. The initial February 10 meeting was postponed a week. So far, in our dealings with the PRC and the Office of Superintendent of Insurance, we have received little support except from Joe Castellano. He had earned our trust. I rationalized, *If Joe says we should do it, then that's what we should do.*

When we arrived at Commissioner Baca's office, she welcomed us with open arms and a kiss on the cheek. I had met other politicians who seemed like straw-stuffed suits, but Shirley was genuine and refreshing. Other politicians we spoke to on both sides of the aisle had turned their heads and closed their eyes or spoken up in false anger and refused to act.

Shirley was a petite woman standing barely five feet tall. Educated and savvy in the Santa Fe arena, she invited us into her office and explained with whom we were really fighting. "Let me tell you what I know about Eric Serna," she said. "He was instrumental in Bill Richardson's run for Congress in 1982. Without Serna's help, an outsider like Richardson didn't stand a chance."

"Wow. Does he really have that much influence?" I asked.

"In the northern part of the state, yes. Serna's extended family has deep roots in almost every part of the state. That, coupled with his relationship with Governor Richardson and Attorney General Patricia Madrid, makes him virtually untouchable. That's why no one wanted to get involved the last time you came up. No one who wants to remain prominent in the state's Democratic Party will step on the governor's toes. That means no one wants to step on Serna's toes. He uses his position as the regulatory authority for the insurance industry to solicit campaign contributions inconspicuously for the governor. And Richardson would not be pleased if his little bank was exposed."

Robert and I couldn't believe that Governor Richardson may have been indirectly behind the denials. It did explain why every other politician and virtually every Santa Fe and Albuquerque attorney had refused to help us, though.

After we met with Shirley, Robert and I walked down the hall to attend the PRC meeting. The interior of the chamber resembled a small courtroom. The walls were covered in wood paneling, and bench seats that resembled church pews were separated into two sides. The bench for the PRC chair was located in the front center of the room and matched the wood. On either side of the chair's bench were lower benches where the remaining commissioners sat. Behind the bench hung the flags of the United States and the state of New Mexico, and situated on the wall in between the flags was the state seal of New Mexico.

After the commission entered and took their seats, the meeting commenced. Robert and I waited patiently while other topics were discussed by the commissioners and concerned citizens who attended the meeting. Soon the topic turned to Eric Serna as he addressed the commission. This is the official transcript of the PRC work session held on February 17, 2005:

> Thank you for the opportunity to respond to the concerns that were raised in your January 31 letter... Con Alma's grants promote systemic outcome motivated change to complement federal, state, tribal, and local government health programs... All citizens, including corporate insurance citizens, have participated in various ways to solve the health crisis in New Mexico. Whether it be through voluntary charitable contribution, or participation in efforts to shape public health care policy through the Governor's Health Care Task Force Initiative, of which I am a member, appointed by him, or the longstanding work of the New Mexico Health and Human Services Committee. I would also add that since the creation of Con Alma, including the $1 million plus in grants that we provided this year, we also provided the

previous two years a total of $1.3 million, making the total $2,300,000, which we have granted throughout the state. In each of your districts, there has been a substantial amount of grants allowed . . .

Robert and I took this to mean, "I am in control of the insurance division. The contributions from insurance companies are voluntary, and I make sure money gets sent to your districts." It came across as a threatening bribe.

Serna continued:

> As to my role as president of the Con Alma Foundation, let me reiterate that I receive no compensation from the Con Alma Health Foundation. I do not actively solicit donations from the insurance industry that I regulate as Superintendent. . . . I ensure that a check is written to the Public Regulation Commission every year to more than cover any possible phone expenses . . . The amount more than compensates this commission and the state for any use of the phone . . . I would never permit a conflict of interest to affect my work and decisions as superintendent of insurance . . . Either party, whether the managed health care plan or the covered person, may raise a conflict of interest and may object at any time throughout the process against an external review panelist or myself . . . As such, I tend to adopt and give substantial deference to the

panel's recommended decision without question, unless there is a substantial legal basis brought to my attention.

Commissioner Baca attempted to condemn Serna. She pointed out that the Governmental Conduct Act, 10-16-3I, states in part, "No public employee may request or receive or offer money, a thing of value or promise thereof that is given in exchange for a promised performance of an official act." She said that Superintendent Serna was in a position of power over a large percentage of contributors and that there was a perception of undue influence. The Act provides that "efforts shall be made to avoid undue influence and abuse of office in public service."

At the end of the meeting, Robert addressed the panel.

> The superintendent reminded all of you that your constituents are receiving money from Con Alma. You, as commissioners, should take note of that when discussing the actions, intention, and the attitude of the superintendent. You must remain impartial and not be bullied or influenced by him.

After his presentation, Eric Serna left the meeting. Robert and I stayed to thank Shirley for sticking up for us, and then we walked toward Joe's office to discuss the meeting and the letter we had received from Jason Marks. We saw Joe standing at the door to Eric's office, engaged in a heated debate.

"I don't care if I can retire in six months," Joe was saying. "I won't do that. You'll just have to fire me, then."

We walked past and continued to Joe's office. A few moments later, Joe walked in with a big grin. I'm not sure if he had seen us pass by, but it seemed like a huge weight had been lifted from his spirit.

Joe said, "The play by Marks is just a ploy to take the heat off of Serna. The commission is giving him a way out while at the same time giving the appearance of firm control of the superintendent—in essence, washing their hands while nothing changes. But as arrogant as Serna is, he'll probably refuse the offer."

A few days after we met with Shirley, Robert went to Roswell, New Mexico, to talk to a longtime family friend[2] who was a prominent businessperson and Democratic fundraiser. Robert told me he felt confident he could get a better feel for what we were up against if we asked our friend to call Governor Richardson on our behalf.

At our friend's office, Robert broke down in tears and explained our situation. Without a word, our friend picked up the phone and hit speed dial. After a moment, our friend left a message: "Eric, you need to call me ASAP to discuss the Maloney appeal."

After a little more discussion, Robert was told to head home and wait for a call. It was a long, stressful trip back to Albuquerque, and he wondered if this could be the answer. Later that evening, our friend called and spoke to Robert, saying, "I'm sorry, but the only thing that will save your wife is a phone call from Governor Richardson to Eric, and I don't have the power to make that

---

[2] Although I was not asked to withhold the name of the family friend, I do not have permission to use the person's name and will not confirm any suspicions about who he or she is.

happen. Your best bet is Bobby Mayfield. You have an excellent attorney."

Robert and I were devastated but hearing that increased our resolve to continue the fight. Shirley worked on gaining the support of two other commissioners in an effort to remove Serna from office. Her insistence began a fracturing of the PRC. The investigative story in the newspaper about Con Alma had sent politicians scrambling to cover their involvement with Con Alma and Eric Serna.

Behind the scenes, our lawsuit against Lovelace and the superintendent of insurance was filed in district court. We never wanted to go to court. All we wanted was to receive what Lovelace was legally obligated to provide in our policy: my bone marrow transplant. In fact, on January 6, 2005, our attorneys sent Lovelace a peace offering:

> Thus far Bill Webber, Joel Newton, and I have spent over $50,000 in attorney's fees. We can and will waive them if and only if this matter can be resolved immediately . . . When Bill, Joel, and I were asked to help Mrs. Maloney, we agreed to take steps to correct what we considered to be fundamentally unjust and rationally indefensible positions by Lovelace Sandia that her bone marrow transplant was simultaneously "medically necessary" yet "experimental." Before filing suit, Bill Webber wrote Lovelace Sandia's counsel a letter virtually begging Lovelace Sandia to do the right thing and give Mrs. Maloney the benefit of the "gray area" into which Lovelace Sandia's

medical director admitted this coverage case falls. With no response to this letter, we began working up the case in earnest . . . Accordingly, we make one final effort to settle this matter before having to resort to the long haul in court . . . The Maloneys hereby offer to dismiss their claims with prejudice, and her counsel agrees to waive all attorney's fees . . .

They did not even have the decency to respond to this second request. Instead, Lovelace opted to wait for the first hearing.

Eleven

Betrayed

I was very ill in November of 2004. The trip to our first court hearing in Santa Fe, just fifty miles away, caused me to wince with every jolt over uneven pavement. I also had huge anxiety and doubts about the court proceedings. The only relief I felt came from Robert's caring and determined demeanor.

"They have to help," Robert said. "Any judge who sees you will understand the urgency."

"I'm feeling weaker every day."

Robert reached over and took my hand. "We have to show the judge that every moment counts. Once he sees the evidence, he'll have to make Lovelace pay for the transplant."

When Robert and I arrived in Santa Fe, we weren't sure how to get to the courthouse. The grid of Santa Fe is a maze of narrow streets that seem to circle through the city, and the traffic is a cluster of confusion. Navigating through the city is complicated by the splendor of the old Southwest architecture. Drivers can't help it when they are distracted by the beauty of the stone Catholic churches and the huge, round building at the center of New Mexico's government.

Robert managed to find the First Judicial District Court on the edge of downtown. He was frustrated because finding a parking space seemed impossible. Our hearing was going to start in less than ten minutes, and the only space he could find was in front of the post office, across the street from the courthouse. The parking was reserved for drivers with postal business. Robert parked in a handicapped spot. "I think we'll be okay. I can't see them towing away a car with a handicap sticker."

At the entrance to the court was a metal detector manned by two sheriff's deputies. We passed through and went to the information kiosk to see where Judge Garcia's courtroom was. When we entered the courtroom, Bill, Bob, and Joel were seated at the counsel table on the left, and another group was seated on the right. I probably looked like the walking dead, with my frail, tiny body hunched over and my face contorted by pain. The lawyers hardly acknowledged me. They glanced over and then returned to their internal conversation.

The judge's bench had a stately presence in front of the carved, wooden seal of New Mexico, and an American flag and a New Mexico flag flanked it. As if that weren't enough to engender reverence and fear, there were wood-paneled walls and curved wooden benches behind the counsel tables.

Joel stood up and walked over to us. "So glad you made it. I was getting worried you would miss the hearing."

"You know how difficult driving in Santa Fe can be," Robert replied.

Joel shook our hands. "Follow me. You can sit behind us."

Bill and Bob greeted us with warm smiles and handshakes. "This shouldn't take long," Bob said. "It looks like we sure got their attention, though. Look at how many lawyers Lovelace and the superintendent of insurance brought to the hearing."

Just then, the bailiff walked in and announced, "All rise."

When you spend much of your time confined to a wheelchair and every move you make causes radiating pain, you become aware of how "All rise" sounds. In church, it's common for the pastor or a lector to say, "Please rise if you are able." I realize that "All rise" is a traditional command in a court of law, but just think about how that command sounds to someone with the pain I've described, possibly *ad nauseum*, to this point in our story.

Everyone stood up. A slender man with a kind face, dressed in a black robe, entered through the door behind the bench. The judge appointed to our case was Timothy Garcia. He was not the original judge assigned to our case. On the advice of a fourth lawyer named David Garza, Bob had asked that our case be reassigned to Judge Garcia. Garza was to be the eyes and ears up north for Bob because of the 300-mile distance between Santa Fe and Las Cruces.

The hearing began. Robert and I listened as our lawyers, Lovelace's lawyers, Eric Serna's lawyer for the Office of Superintendent of Insurance, and Judge Garcia conversed in legalese. After just a few minutes, the bailiff again said, "All rise."

Everyone stood up, and Judge Garcia left the bench and exited through the same door behind his bench.

As our attorneys turned around, Robert blurted out: "You didn't even bring up the tape of Cigna closing our file three days before the superintendent ruled."

"I understand how you feel," Joel answered. "Let's step out into the hall and discuss it further."

The hearing was disappointing because no evidence was allowed, a far cry from what Robert and I had envisioned from watching television. But Judge Garcia did agree to an expedited hearing agenda for our case. Bob told us we had obtained our first victory in court. It seemed that moving forward quickly with the case would be possible, and the race against the clock in the courts had begun.

Our attorneys were pleased with how the proceedings had gone and felt that they could have a fair trial in Santa Fe after all. Northern New Mexico attorney David Garza had expressed concern that three southern New Mexico attorneys might have a tough go in Santa Fe, so Bob had decided to bring Garza in as a fourth attorney for our case. Robert and I had never met him.

A few weeks later, we had our second court hearing. Bob explained that this could go very quickly. As he put it, "Once the judge allows us to depose Eric Serna, Lovelace, and the superintendent will beg for a settlement and agree to pay for Zelphoe's treatment." Bob reasoned that Serna would have to plead the fifth or risk incriminating himself and Lovelace officials in criminal activity centered in the Con Alma scandal.

At the next hearing, Judge Garcia refused to rule on any of the motions our attorneys had proposed. Joel gave a presentation using well-designed poster-style cards, but the Judge seemed unimpressed by the facts and unsuccessfully tried to cover his laugh under his breath. In fact, Judge Garcia asserted that Bill was asking him to waive our common law and statutory claims in an attempt to expedite the proceedings. Bob assured the judge that in no way was he attempting to waive any claims. The judge told our attorneys to rethink their case closely before the next hearing.

As we left the building, Bill Webber shook his head. "It looks like we might have gotten snookered right out of the gate. I thought I knew Garza pretty well. He told us to recuse the first judge. He said Judge Garcia was who we wanted."

"He didn't even show up," Joel responded. "I want Garza off this case. I don't care if we have to drive up for every hearing; at least we won't have to worry about who to trust."

Mayfield looked up the steps at the courthouse entrance. "I've never seen anything like it. I could tell by the judge's facial expressions that he understood everything, and right when I thought he was going to make a ruling, he went on to another topic. This should have been an open-and-shut case on getting Serna's deposition."

Just then, opposing counsel Nelson Franse stepped out of the courthouse, beaming and adjusting his glasses. He walked down the steps past Webber, Newton, and Mayfield, then stopped and turned to them. I could feel Robert's arm tense up.

In a smug tone, Franse remarked, "I don't know about you guys, but I like this judge."

Franse's attitude drew a line in the sand—a line everyone involved on our side was determined to cross. Looking back, I reflect on the integrity our lawyers displayed, and it brings comfort knowing that not all lawyers can be dumped into the same basket. On the other hand, it appeared that David Garza had been against us from the beginning. His recommendation to accept Judge Garcia would have dire consequences. Years later, Bill Webber told me he encountered Garza in front of the courthouse in Santa Fe. The two locked eyes and Garza said, "I hope you understand."

Twelve

Sabotage

Late in 2004, Robert and I learned that there were four fronts in the battle to save my life: legal, media, political, and medical. On the legal and medical side, Lovelace argued that I was not a viable candidate for the stem cell transplant; Robert and I had to prove I was a good candidate for the procedure. Dr. Frank O'Sullivan had asserted this point vigorously.

One day, when Robert drove me to a routine doctor visit at O'Sullivan's clinic, there was something different about my physician's demeanor. He seemed distant yet asked very direct questions. "You've lost another five pounds. I'm not sure what to try next. How's your appeal going?"

My husband did not pick up on the change in attitude and responded in a normal way: "It doesn't look good. We're in court now, and Lovelace is disputing my wife's eligibility for the transplant."

"That might be correct. I just heard back from Dr. Traynor. It seems . . . Gabrielle is not a candidate for the stem cell transplant, after all."

Robert and I were at a loss for words. We left O'Sullivan's office, unsure what would happen. Robert later told me what he did next. Once we returned home, he called Ann Traynor to verify that I had been dropped from the stem cell program. It was true. Traynor explained her reasoning for dropping me: My rheumatologist had informed her that I had only kidney problems and that no other organs were affected by the lupus.

Robert was outraged. He shot back, "That is not true! Her lupus is affecting her kidneys, lungs, heart, intestines, and brain. Did Dr. O'Sullivan send you her records?"

Traynor had received only some basic blood work and a referral from O'Sullivan. She told Robert that based on the involvement of multiple organs, I *was* a candidate for the transplant after all. She apologized and recommended that we seek Dr. Yu Oyama at Northwestern University in Chicago for a second opinion. She also suggested changing my current doctor. I knew Robert was furious, but what he did next I did not discover until years later.

Betrayal is an ugly thing. It can deflate your enthusiasm, or it can ignite a fire. After sitting in the waiting room for almost an hour to get a response to his request to see O'Sullivan, Robert stormed into his office. I'm not sure what Robert told him, but the doctor got the message. The doctor's medical notes after that encounter read:

> Mrs. Maloney's husband came into my office this morning. He was visibly upset about Dr. Traynor's

refusal to accept Mrs. Maloney for the stem cell transplant. I think he fired me. Mr. Maloney said he was taking Mrs. Maloney to another specialist in El Paso, I believe. I will wait for further communication from them.

Needless to say, we had no further contact with him except at his deposition years later.

After this incident, it became difficult to obtain new doctors in the Lovelace network. Doctors talk to each other, and the fact that I had an open lawsuit against Lovelace undermined my ability to secure needed specialists. I heard excuses like, "The doctor will be out of town," or "The doctor is not seeing new patients." The attitude at Lovelace had changed dramatically.

I needed to go out of network to receive medical attention from several specialists. The nephrologist I chose was very professional. I also got a new rheumatologist. He reviewed my history and asked if I would do a kidney biopsy. The nephrologist told me there was no need for the biopsy because the damage to my kidneys was already done.

The rheumatologist was persistent, but I was reluctant and reminded him that the nephrologist insisted my kidneys were doomed to fail. He countered that the damage might be temporary and might subside if my lupus was brought under control. The nephrologist gave Robert, and me hope that he might be able to save my kidneys. He wanted to look for another reason for my decreased kidney function other than lupus or IVIG that could be corrected. I was willing to grasp any hope.

On the day of the biopsy, I had doubts about the procedure.

The words of the nephrologist echoed in my head: *The damage is already done.*

Robert tried to be encouraging: "It's a simple biopsy. Besides, if it helps the doctor save your kidneys even for a few years, it's worth it."

This was not my first kidney biopsy. I had undergone the grueling, hour-long outpatient procedure once years before.

After I got into my gown, I was placed on a stretcher and wheeled down the hall. Robert followed. We pushed past the swinging doors and into a room with a bright light and monitoring equipment. Once in the procedure room, I was rolled over on my stomach and felt lidocaine being applied to numb the area. Robert held my hand as the doctor used ultrasound to locate my kidney. Then Robert had to step back.

A dull pressure moved slightly on my skin, and then a sharp pain pierced my back. I began to cry, and Robert moved closer to comfort me.

After the procedure was finished, the doctor said, "Let's make sure we have enough tissue for testing." I watched as another person dressed in scrubs pushed the biopsy material from the needle into a clear container.

After a moment the doctor told the assistant, "It looks like you missed." The doctor apologized to me for the mistake and said he needed another sample.

I braced for another try. The dull pressure moved in a small, circular motion as I tensed up. This time, the pain grew severe—like a piece of me was being ripped from my back. I couldn't hold back the tears. Robert hugged me, and after several more tries, we heard, "Looks like we have enough." It was over. I could go home.

But my blood pressure spiked, and the pain intensified. The doctor ordered the nurse to move me to an observation room. After a few moments, I felt faint, and the doctor ordered pain medication.

When I returned to dialysis the next day, I felt life draining out of me. The dialysis center doctor ordered a sonogram of my kidney after I informed him of the biopsy the day before. The biopsy had caused severe internal bleeding. I was hospitalized for several days; relief finally came when a doctor removed the lost blood from the kidney.

In the end, the new biopsy did not show any hope for recovery of my kidney function. In fact, a second doctor told me the procedure was unnecessary, just as the nephrologist had. I later discovered that the new rheumatologist was friends with Frank O'Sullivan and had once worked at Lovelace. I can't help but wonder if he ordered the biopsy to try to prove that my kidney function was not as bad as it was after O'Sullivan ordered certain treatments or because of the lawsuit his colleague was part of.

I did not see that particular rheumatologist again. In fact, when I called to set up an appointment, his receptionist told me I needed to find another rheumatologist because he was retiring. He did not retire. No doubt, he was worried because of the complications of the biopsy, involving admitted mistakes. He may have also dropped me because he had done what he could to try and help his friend, Frank O'Sullivan.

The nephrologist also dropped me as a patient and assigned me to a colleague. I understood he was angry that I had gone against his recommendation not to get the kidney biopsy, but I was hanging on to any hope of a life without dialysis. I didn't realize how severe a risk the rheumatologist had created for me.

I replaced both rheumatologists with a general practitioner for my basic needs, such as prescriptions and referrals. He ended up being a good person, but he fell short as a physician. He stuck with me until I moved from Albuquerque. He was later deposed about my condition and treatment while under Lovelace's care, and his oversight was brought into question by one of our lawyers, who suggested we include him in the lawsuit. But I couldn't in good conscience sue this doctor. He had been willing to take me, even though he was not a specialist when other Lovelace doctors avoided me. Even people who just want to help can sometimes make mistakes, and I am grateful for this doctor and his wonderful nurse, who not only looked after my physical needs but also helped me emotionally. I am sorry he had to endure such a brutal deposition.

Thirteen

Adding Insult to Injury

A deposition is a sworn question-and-answer session done outside the courtroom, but it carries the same weight as court testimony. The deposition I did in March 2005, before I left to receive my stem cell transplant in October 2005, could have been my last plea to the court—a final farewell.

In fact, Joel Newton asked as the deposition commenced, "You know why I'm doing your deposition today, don't you?"

"Because I might not come back from Chicago alive."

Mine was the first deposition agreed upon by the defense and Judge Garcia. Robert and I met Joel at the office of the Rodey Law Firm, which occupied two floors at the top of one of the tallest buildings in Albuquerque. It sat in the middle of downtown and offered views beyond the city limits from any window. We passed opulently decorated conference rooms on the way to meet Nelson Franse, who would be representing Lovelace for the deposition.

When we entered his office, Franse stood up and shook hands with Joel, but he ignored Robert and me. After an uncomfortable twenty seconds, Robert, like the gentleman he is, walked up to Franse and shook his hand. After that, Franse said hello to me in a forced polite way. Robert later told me Joel believed that Franse wanted us to meet at the Rodey Law Office so they could intimidate us with the size, money, and status their law firm projected. If that was his intent, he failed. Rather than being intimidated, I was determined. This was my chance to tell the world how I had witnessed Lovelace encouraging doctors to limit medical options for their patients. I believe Lovelace executives received inflated compensation at the expense of human lives.

Franse's office was large enough to accommodate the deposition, as were the conference rooms we had passed on our way in. Yet he escorted us to a repurposed storage closet. A long, narrow table surrounded by office chairs occupied the center. At each end of the room were doors to hallways. As we entered, everyone had a hard time squeezing past the chairs to take a seat. At one end of the table sat the court reporter, ready to transcribe my deposition.

Once we were seated and I was sworn in, Joel Newton asked, "Are you feeling up to answering questions today?" All eyes in the room were on me. That is every eye except the two behind the bright red, seventies-throwback glasses of Nelson Franse. I paused and watched as Franse kicked his boots up on the table across from me, took a sports magazine from his briefcase, raised it to cover his face, and began to flip through it as if I were not in the room. Joel kept asking me questions, occasionally looking at Franse, who continued skimming his magazine.

I felt like crying as I answered Joel's questions, not only from the sting of remembering the inhumane care Lovelace had provided but also from the pain in my joints.

Franse seemed to ignore the entire first half of the deposition. After Joel finished he then asked Franse if he had any questions for me before we took a break. As I remember, without even looking away from the magazine, he said one word: "Nope." He closed the magazine and slid it across the table before standing up. "I guess that wraps this half up." The court reporter took a few seconds to finish typing as Franse walked out of the room and down the hall. Joel and Bill discussed Franse's demeanor while Robert and I took a break to encourage one another before the second half began.

After a few minutes, Franse returned to the room and said, "Let's get this wrapped up quickly. I have an important meeting."

I could sense Robert's anger as he tensed up and then breathed out slowly. He encouraged me to focus on the deposition, not Franse. I looked pathetic on the outside, but my mind was stern and ready for battle.

The court reporter said, "We're on the record," and the deposition resumed.

Joel sat across from me and continued to offer comforting smiles as Franse, the former University of New Mexico Lobo starting forward, launched his callous assault.

"Are you saying that Lovelace doesn't care if you live or die, Mrs. Maloney?" he asked.

"Their actions speak for themselves," I answered. "I don't need to add to them."

"It seems that you were not happy with the panel's decision. Do you think Lovelace bribed the panel?"

"I don't know what Lovelace did."

"Do you think Lovelace should pay for the transplant because you think it is covered in the insurance contract, and it doesn't matter to you what the contract says? Is that correct?"

"I have a health insurance policy that covers my health. I expect it to pay for my health care."

"If the contract says it is not covered, should the insurance pay?"

Franse continued his assault to make me either lose my temper or succumb to guilt. But I had no part of it either. On occasion, Joel objected to some questions, but for the most part, I went on a verbal toe-to-toe with the basketball giant as he pounded the relevance of the insurance contract into the record. As abruptly as Franse began his intimidation, he ended it. He looked at his watch and walked out of the room. Joel reinforced Robert's opinion that I had handled myself with courageous dignity, although I had felt like a little girl on the playground waiting for the school bully to throw mud in my face. We all stopped the discussion when Franse's secretary walked in and said, "Mr. Franse asked me to show you out."

Robert and I took this encounter as a blatant message from Lovelace: "We have no reason to take you seriously." The fact that Judge Garcia had prevented us from obtaining depositions from Eric Serna and top Lovelace officials, combined with the careless attitude of Lovelace, the Rodey Law Firm, and Nelson Franse, and the comments our family friend had made about the governor's involvement, solidified our determination to continue the lawsuit.

It would be a long shot, but it was our only shot. Robert and our attorneys worried that Lovelace's calculated tactics would delay any relief that would save my life. I was afraid the process would take too long, but watching how the people around me were dedicated to my survival gave me the courage to fight on.

Fourteen

Assaulted, and Again

During the time of the denial and the lawsuit, in mid-2005, I was hospitalized several times. One time, I was lying in bed with an IV drip connected to my arm. Robert had just left to grab something to eat and said he would be back in a couple of hours. The patient in the next room was screaming for someone to come, but no one responded. I looked at the clock next to the bed. It was two o'clock in the morning. I was afraid.

The door slowly opened, and I sighed with relief when I thought I saw Robert. The lady next door had fallen silent, and something didn't seem right. The figure paused at the door. I strained to verify that it was Robert, but the light was too dim. Slowly, the figure moved closer.

"Robert?" I whispered.

As the figure continued to approach, my eyes opened wide. I tried to scoot away. The visitor appeared to be a large male orderly. He leaned over me and put one hand over my mouth. His breath stank of cigarettes. I twitched and then froze as he reached between my legs with his other hand. I struggled as best I could, trying to shake my head enough to uncover my mouth and scream, but he pressed harder. He began pulling down my panties and then stopped. The sound of someone pushing a cart down the hall startled him. He let go of my panties and put his finger to his lips, ordering me to be silent. Then he leaned over and licked my cheek with his cigarette tongue. He motioned again for me to be silent and released the pressure of his hand from my mouth. I was too afraid to scream. As he left the room, I gasped for air. I lay motionless, silently crying, until Robert came.

I was ashamed, and most women would relate to that feeling. An incident like this is not the woman's fault, but when she looks into the eyes of the one she loves and knows she has been touched by someone else, shame is a normal feeling. It was a struggle for me to tell Robert. He immediately notified the floor nurse who called security. Later that morning, a social worker came to take my statement. She was more concerned that my medication had caused delusions than she was about finding out who had assaulted me. Robert voiced outrage, but all the social worker said was that they would "look into it." To this day, the scent of cigarettes sends a chill down my spine.

The period between early 2004 and the end of 2007 was by far the most devastating and uncertain time in my life. When you are sick, some people view you as a target. It's like a coyote stalking a crippled deer: As soon as she is apart from the herd, she is a victim.

At a time when I didn't know whom to trust, an older woman befriended me. At first, she was someone who listened well, and she got along with our children. She was what you would expect a young grandmother to be. We sometimes went to lunch or spent time at each other's homes.

On one occasion, Robert needed to be out of town for a night. After a brief discussion, we decided that the twins and I should stay at my new friend's house. Later that evening, at about ten o'clock, I put the twins to sleep in her guest room and returned to the living room to watch television. A few moments later, the woman walked out of her bedroom and asked, "Would you like a soda?" I accepted the offer, and she went to the kitchen and returned, handing me a glass. When I took a sip, the soda seemed a bit flat, and the taste was off. I thought it must be from the bottom of a two-liter bottle of generic cola. I didn't want to come across as rude or ungrateful, so I drank the soda. The woman took the empty glass and put it in the kitchen before returning to her bedroom. I soon became drowsy and started fading in and out. I'm not sure about the time, but at one point, I heard other people in the house talking but couldn't keep my eyes open.

In the morning, when I woke up on the couch, my head was pounding. I knew something wasn't right, and I was sore in places I should not have been—private places. I struggled to my feet and noticed two strange men walking out the front door. I stumbled down the hall to check on the twins, who were still asleep. The woman seemed to be gone. Images of things that had occurred during the night flooded my mind, and I rushed to the restroom and violently vomited. My defense mechanism kicked in as I tried to convince myself nothing had happened. I woke the children and rushed home.

The next morning, I called the woman. I wanted to get her

on record admitting to what had happened. She seemed afraid and hung up. A few minutes later I received a call from a woman claiming to be a police officer. After mentioning my neighbor, the woman's language turned foul, and she threatened me, telling me to leave her friend alone. I handed the phone to Robert. He listened for a moment and asked, "What is your badge number?" The woman hung up.

Over the next few days, Robert could tell something was disturbing me. Night after night, I woke in a cold sweat as disgusting images haunted my dreams. The guilt multiplied whenever he asked, "Why are you keeping your distance from me? Just tell me what's wrong." Again, I was ashamed.

I have learned to take threats seriously and to act accordingly, but what do you do when the people threatening you have no accountability? Robert called the Albuquerque Police Department to see if the woman was an officer. The name and phone number Robert gave the person on the phone checked out. The obscene lady was, in fact, an officer. Robert and I followed the advice of the person he'd spoken with and went in to file a complaint against her at Internal Affairs. You would have thought we were the criminals! The prevailing attitude was, "How dare you make accusations against the police?"

The woman interviewing me said, "It seems like there's something else troubling you."

I began crying uncontrollably. Robert put his arms around me and tried to comfort me. I was so afraid to tell him what had happened at that woman's house, but I couldn't live with the shame by myself.

The officer said the allegations were serious and left us alone to discuss what kind of action we wanted to take. Robert wanted to press charges, but I wanted to move past this nightmare. Just letting him know what was troubling me had eased some of the stress and frustration. We ultimately decided not to pursue charges, primarily because of the woman's affiliation with the Albuquerque police.

The Albuquerque police had a reputation as renegades who had little oversight. A story in *The New York Times* from April 10, 2014, sums up why we feared the police:

> Too often, the Justice Department said, the officers kicked, punched and violently restrained non-threatening people, and seldom were the officers reprimanded . . . "What we found was a pattern or practice of systemic deficiencies that have pervaded the Albuquerque Police Department for many years," Jocelyn Samuels, acting assistant attorney general for the department's civil rights division, said at a news conference on Thursday.
>
> The Albuquerque police, she said, suffered from "inadequate oversight, inadequate investigation of incidents of force, inadequate training of officers to ensure they understand what is permissible or not." As a result the Police Department had engaged "in a pattern or practice of violating residents' Fourth Amendment rights in an unconstitutional manner," Mrs. Samuels said.

A mutual acquaintance later told me the woman was being investigated for possessing child pornography. By that time, the cynic in me was getting stronger and I could only think, "No wonder she took such an interest in my children."

Fifteen

A Promise of Hope

I had one shot to persuade a doctor who didn't know me that I was the right candidate for his life-saving treatment. Fear and anxiety gripped me the entire week leading up to my trip to visit Dr. Yu Oyama at Northwestern University in Chicago. I spent every waking hour thinking of how to convey why he should choose me and wondering if Lovelace was sabotaging my attempt behind the scenes.

In contrast, Robert was optimistic. He continued with his work, taking care of the children and me even though I knew we were drowning financially. If he was anxious or worried, he hid it well. Robert had pulled out our last $2,000 to pay for airfare, a one-night hotel stay, and the initial interview and tests, which cost almost $1,300. When we landed in Chicago on Thursday, December 16, 2004, we had a $100 bill, and I had a hundred reasons flowing through my mind why I would be rejected.

A few weeks earlier, I had secretly sent Oyama all the medical records I could get from Lovelace. Instead of asking Northwestern to request them, I requested them for personal use to hide the fact that Oyama was going to evaluate me. Robert and I planned the trip to Chicago without the knowledge of any of my Albuquerque doctors. This was my last chance at life, and I was not willing to let another Lovelace doctor sabotage it by withholding information from the transplant doctor.

Oyama reviewed my medical records and approved me for the evaluation. On November 9, 2004, he wrote a letter to Lovelace. I have no recollection of Lovelace responding to this letter, nor have I found any evidence that Lovelace responded to the doctor's request in any of my extensive research, except for a letter referenced in the next chapter.

> To Whom It May Concern:
>
> Mrs. Zelphoe Maloney is a 39-year-old female who has been suffering from systemic lupus erythematosus (SLE) with kidney involvement. Her disease has failed therapies including corticosteroids, cyclophosphamide and various other agents. Her renal disease has progressed to WHO class III/IV on renal biopsy. We are requesting permission for evaluation at Northwestern for treatment of her refractory disease.
>
> Our stem cell transplantation has been helping patients with severe SLE who failed conventional

therapies. Our program started in 1997, and we have performed this therapy for 46 patients with life-threatening refractory lupus and had minimal mortality and morbidity. At Northwestern University, we have the largest number of cases and lead the world in this field. We have tremendous expertise and skills in treatment of severe autoimmune diseases with stem cell transplantation.

Once Mrs. Maloney is evaluated and determined as a candidate, we should proceed with the transplant as soon as possible in order to improve outcome. I believe that the therapy will help her condition and provide long-term benefit compared to conventional therapies.

Sincerely,

Yu Oyama, MD

Being at Northwestern Memorial Hospital in Chicago was like being in a foreign city. When we got out of the cab in front of the massive building, we were already lost. The temperature on Friday, December 17, was in the low 20s, and our breath misted in the moist air before dissipating in the breeze.

Robert rushed me out of the cold through the first door we saw. Smiling hospital staff at the information desk let us know we were in the wrong tower. We needed to hurry to the other one across the street if we were going to make the appointment on time, but hurrying meant shooting pain in my legs. But we did it. We made our first appointment with just seconds to spare. In this section of the hospital, buildings stood over twenty stories tall and took up entire city blocks. Outlying facilities were scattered all around the main hospital in smaller buildings. I remember seeing another tower under construction a couple of blocks away. It would eventually become the Northwestern Women's Hospital. At that time, only part of the steel frame was complete, and gigantic cranes dominated the scene as they moved steel beams high into the air.

Our first appointment was on the fourteenth floor with Dr. Yu Oyama—or so we thought. Once we checked in, we began filling out multiple forms. Then, we were sent to several other offices for tests that took all morning. As the day progressed, my anxiety peaked. I could tell my blood pressure was increasing dramatically, and my eyes felt swollen.

After our last test, we had just under an hour before our next appointment, so we decided to go to the hospital's dining area. On the way, the tension welled up in me, and I began to cry. Robert hugged me, but I began to hyperventilate. Robert had to help me pace myself until I could breathe normally.

My wonderful husband then took my hand and started to pray. I closed my eyes and pictured my children playing at home together, and a sense of peace filled my heart. Robert wrapped his arms around me and asked, "Do you feel better now?" At that point, I reached deep within for strength as I realized my love for my family had increased beyond what I had ever thought possible. I nodded.

After lunch, we went back to Oyama's office. Our appointment with him was not until 2:30, but we were to meet with his nurse, Kim Young, at 1:30.

My anxiety began to creep back as we waited for Kim to come into the exam room. I had spoken to her on numerous occasions as she guided me through the process of requesting to be part of the research Northwestern was conducting.

When she entered the room, her smile, and cheerful demeanor blended with her soft-spoken words. "I am so delighted you made it," she said. "How was your flight?"

My anxiety subsided. "It was long, but I'm grateful to be here. I just hope I'm accepted."

"Well, if there is any way, Dr. Oyama will find it. You're in good hands. Now let me explain what the transplant entails."

Kim offered a lot of comfort in her explanation and answered our questions with gentle confidence—not a hint of condescension or arrogance. What a change of tone from what Robert and I had become accustomed to with Lovelace. Kim explained how my "mother cells" would be harvested from my bone marrow. My old immune system would be reduced to as close to zero as possible, and the harvested cells would be reintroduced and begin establishing a healthy immune system. I had no doubt she knew this procedure inside and out. Not only did she know it, she believed in it, and her belief was contagious.

By the end of our hour-long interview, Robert and I were relatively at ease with the procedure, even though Kim reminded us, albeit abruptly, of the possibility of the transplant being fatal.

She asked if we had any more questions to discuss before Dr. Oyama came in. Robert asked about patients who had already received the transplant: "How are they doing?"

She answered, "Dr. Oyama and Dr. Richard Burt, the pioneer of the program, have helped many people who had no other treatment, including people with lupus and multiple sclerosis. Almost eighty percent have seen remission and are now living substantially better lives. I have a list of patients who have volunteered to speak with anyone who would like a first-hand conversation about the program. I think the woman from Florida would be a perfect match for you. She is a young mother like you. Would you like to contact her?"

"Of course! That is so kind of her to offer to share her experience."

Kim convinced Robert and me that the transplant was our best hope. Although we didn't realize it at the time, Kim Young was to become our guide to survival.

I can laugh about it now, but when Dr. Yu Oyama walked into the exam room, for a moment I doubted his ability to help me. Don't get me wrong—I was grateful to be there—but he looked nothing like what I expected of a doctor pioneering a breakthrough medical treatment. Oyama was not the seventy-year-old, white-haired, reserved man with glasses I had expected, but rather a young, black-haired, friendly, funny, vibrant individual who seemed to be in his twenties. In reality, he was thirty-seven.

We bonded immediately. His caring demeanor and concerned questions left me with no doubt that he was determined to help. Yu Oyama felt like a brother to me. In fact, my brother is a pediatrician and displayed similar qualities and compassion toward me. By the time we finished our interview, I had no doubt this man would save my life. If I'd had any strength left, I would have jumped for joy.

There was one possible setback. The decision was not Oyama's alone. He needed the approval of multiple specialists, including a cardiologist, pulmonologist, nephrologist, and rheumatologist. Although Oyama's demeanor was optimistic, he did express concern about my condition. According to the medical records he received, it appeared that Lovelace had caused my health to deteriorate by allowing only one doctor to manage my care. I should have been seeing several specialists in the fields of those now deciding my fate.

Oyama stayed with us, answering all our questions. In fact, he stayed more than an hour, which I found comfortingly strange for a doctor. At Lovelace, the maximum time a doctor would visit was about fifteen minutes.

After the appointment, Robert and I rushed downstairs. Our flight back to Albuquerque was at 4:50 p.m., and it was 3:45. Robert took my hand as we hurried out of the hospital. Immediately, he started flagging down a cab to take us to the airport.

"I'm sorry, hon, but we can't miss this flight," he compassionately explained. He tried to play it off with a smile, but I knew if we missed the flight, we would be sleeping at the airport until we could catch another one. All of our credit cards had been canceled, and the debit card we had tied to our checking account was overdrawn. Another night in a hotel was not an option.

We made it to the gate with no time to spare. As the plane took off, I looked out the window at the lights of Chicago and thought, *I'll be back.*

Sixteen

Reach for the Moon

It was Thursday, December 23, 2004. Robert and I were out looking for Christmas presents for our five children. We were hopeful that some stores would offer big discounts this late in the season. We had less than $150 to purchase five gifts, and I felt horrible. Our business had always provided for us in the past, but the cost of covering the expenses of my condition had "stolen Christmas"—or at least, that was how I felt.

As we were walking through Toys-R-Us, Robert's phone rang. He answered and, after a pause, said, "Yes, Kim, she's here with me."

My heart began racing, and I grabbed Robert's hand and squeezed. This was the call I had been anxiously anticipating and sometimes fearing for the past week. Robert nodded a couple of times but paid no attention to the shoppers who bumped into us as we stood in the middle of the aisle.

Then, a big smile appeared on his face, and he squeezed my hand. I knew before the words came out of his mouth. "You're accepted!" he said. "You can get the transplant."

This was the best news we had received in a very long time. I was so grateful that Dr. Oyama and his staff had wrapped up the gift of life for me. All I needed was Lovelace to hand me the gift. But the gift could expire, and the clock was ticking. Because of my rapidly deteriorating health, soon, the stem cell transplant door would slam shut. It seemed this could be a very special Christmas, and indeed it was. My family and I were hopeful that this would be the last Christmas I would be sick.

What happened next still perplexes me today. I received a letter from Lovelace on January 27, 2005, that was dated January 26, 2005:

> Dear Member:
>
> Lovelace Health Plan has authorized the following service(s):
>
> Request for/to:
>
> Facility name, if applicable: Northwestern Memorial Hospital
>
> Physician name, if applicable: Yu Oyama
>
> Practitioner requested from, if applicable: Frank O'Sullivan

Approved Service(s): Transplant Outpatient (Autolog Stem Cell/BMT)

Authorization #: 91493

Approval period: 12/14/2005-to-12/14/2005

Additional information: Authorization Decisions: Approval 12 Month

When Robert and I read this letter, we thought Lovelace had decided to do the right thing. Cautiously optimistic, we called Bob Mayfield immediately. He asked us to fax him the letter and said he believed it could be in response to the January 23 *Albuquerque Journal* story "Under Fire" about our case and our efforts to raise money from the public for the transplant. Or it might be a response to a letter he had written to Lovelace on January 6:

> We have all come to a crossroads in this case that permits a one-time opportunity for an early resolution.
>
> Before proposing that resolution, let me describe the crossroads:
>
> Zelphoe Maloney has just been accepted for a bone marrow transplant at Northwestern Memorial Hospital in Chicago.

The cost to Northwestern alone could be as little as $75,000 payable up front.

Thus far, Bill Webber, Joel Newton, and I have been willing to assist Zelphoe, without worry about payment. We have spent over $50,000 in attorney's fees. We can and will waive them if and only if this matter can be resolved immediately.

We are all facing motion practice and depositions that will cost more in the next two months than Mrs. Maloney's transplant will cost.

If we cannot resolve this matter now, Mrs. Maloney will be forced to raise funds by publicizing her plight—with uncertain results.

    Bob called us back after reading the letter and said we should prepare to go to Chicago. He was not certain of the wording in the approval letter, but he would call Nelson Franse for clarification. He was hopeful that the offer from Lovelace was sincere.

    I was torn in two. One part of me wanted to scream for joy, but another part grew angry at the thought that this had resembled the first approval I'd received over the phone from Cigna a few months earlier.

    Joel drafted and faxed a letter to Nelson Franse's office immediately.

Dear Carolyn, Max, Zach, Jocelyn, and Nelson,

Enclosed is a letter that Mrs. Maloney received in the mail. It looks like approval for the transplant at Northwestern due to the line in the middle of the page that reads:

"Approved Service(s): Transplant Outpatient (Autolog Stem Cell/BMT)"

I'm confused about the word "Outpatient" and assume it is incorrect. I'm also assuming that the one-day window for "Approved period" is also a typo and that it should be a one-year window.

It appears there has finally been an approval. We simply need clarification of these issues immediately so we can dismiss the judicial appeal and advise the court that there is not a need for an expedited docket.

Please shed some light on this so that we can guide ourselves.

Looking back, it was the uncertainty that troubled me the most. I had come to grips with the fact that I might not survive and had accepted the fact that Lovelace would not relent from its callous treatment. But looking at my children and thinking *I might have decades* and then realizing it might only be months hurt me the most.

The next day, Robert called Bob twice, but Lovelace had not responded to the faxed letter or the phone calls from Bob or Joel. At this point, Robert and I were at our wits' end. We had started making arrangements for the trip, but not wholeheartedly like before. Something didn't seem right, and it was taking its toll on us. The children could sense it. The past twenty-four hours had been a free-for-all as the children did everything they could to get our attention—writing on the walls, screaming, fighting, and refusing to eat. These uncommon behaviors repeated themselves like waves of tension pounding on the shores of my sanity.

On January 28, 2005, I received another letter from Lovelace dated January 27, 2005:

NOTICE OF DENIAL OF MEDICAL COVERAGE

We have denied coverage of the following medical services or items that you or your physician requested: Autologous Stem Cell Bone Marrow Transplant for the treatment of SLE

After review of the information submitted and the terms of your plan benefits, a Health Plan Medical Director/Physician Reviewer denied this request because:

Your health plan considers stem cell transplantation for the treatment of SLE to be an unproven/experimental treatment that is excluded from coverage. There is a lack of evidence in the published, peer-reviewed medical literature to support the safety and efficacy of this procedure for this problem. In addition, the request is to provide this therapy as part of an ongoing clinical trial, which also shows this treatment to be unproven/ experimental.

This determination was based on the following criteria/guideline:

Member Handbook

Decisions related to medical care are your responsibility together with your treating provider, and we recommend that you discus alternative treatment options with him/her.

We regret that this decision is not more favorable.

Lovelace's response was **bold** and *swift*: *"You're on your own!"* This approval and then denial by Lovelace didn't sting as bad as the first time they had done it. I guess I expected it.

Lovelace's continued denials and stalling legal tactics resulted in my continued health deterioration. Nelson Franse appeared to use every opportunity to mock the severity of my situation in the courtroom, even as I sat ten feet from him.

I remember one instance when Bob Mayfield shocked the whole courtroom. It was one of the few times when Franse was caught off guard. Franse had stood up, removed his Elton John-style glasses, and addressed the court: "I understand that Mrs.

Maloney's health is a great issue. I don't think anyone would dispute that. But paying for experiments is not the responsibility of my client."

Bob started to lick his lips; he appeared jittery, about ready to jump from his seat. He was usually calm and collected, but as Franse continued discounting Lovelace's responsibility, Bob sat on the edge of his seat, obviously eager to speak.

He suddenly stood up. After a brief moment of silence, he responded in an angry tone. "We have a third party willing to pay for the transplant, Your Honor! This will allow the question of the timetable to be alleviated. The defense can stop referring to time as an issue for not supplying the discovery, which we humbly request the court to compel Lovelace to provide."

Bob, Joel, and Bill turned around to look at us. Robert stared at our attorneys for a second, then looked back at me and began to cry. As for me, I was stunned. You would think that unbelievable news—someone willing to pay $75,000 for a stranger to receive proper medical treatment—would have changed the dynamic in the courtroom and the way Lovelace and the Rodey Law Firm viewed this case.

But after a moment of stunned silence, Franse looked over at Bob Mayfield, then at the judge, and said, "We need to know the identity of this person and review the relationship he has with the Maloneys and their counsel."

Joel told us the person donating was a modest man who wished to remain anonymous. For a moment I thought, maybe it's someone we know donating the money. Bob explained that he was not at liberty to disclose the identity of the donor to us, and we did not press the issue.

Once again, Franse demanded to know who had offered to pay. Judge Garcia recommended that Bob reveal the individual's identity to the court. Bob stood up and said, "He has asked to remain anonymous but has agreed to be revealed if the defense would use his anonymity to stall my client's treatment." We held our breath as Bob announced, "Frank Borman has made arrangements with the Borman Foundation to pay for the stem cell treatment at Northwestern."

Franse had no objections. Who could object to this famous astronaut's integrity and generosity?

Frank Borman was Commander of Apollo 8, NASA's first successful mission to circle the moon. He also earned NASA's highest honor, the Congressional Space Medal of Honor. His view on humanity is described well in a quote: "When you're finally up on the moon, looking back at the earth, all these differences and nationalistic traits are pretty well going to blend, and you're going to get a concept that maybe this is really one world and why the hell can't we learn to live together like decent people?" (*Newsweek* magazine, December 23, 1968)

We had no idea that Borman and his wife had a special interest in New Mexico and moved to Las Cruces in 2006.

Even now, Robert and I have never met or spoken to Borman. All we are sure of is that Lovelace would have let me die had he not felt compelled to help me, to fill the decency gap Lovelace had created. Bob Mayfield asked Robert and me to meet with Frank Borman, but I couldn't find it in myself to meet him without breaking down into tears, and based on his actions, I understood he was not seeking praise. From my heart and on behalf of my husband and children, I'd like to say, "Thank you is not enough, but thank you, Colonel Borman. You are a true hero."

My husband wrote a poem for me on our twenty-fifth anniversary, something I would not have been able to share with him if not for Frank Borman.

> If you ever doubt me
> If you want to cry
> Go out into the night, my dear
> And look into the sky
> Tell me what you see there
> Shining in the night
> Reach up and grab one,
> Hold with all your might
> For every star that shimmers
> For every one you see
> Is just another year, dear
> I need you here with me
> Forever I will love you
> You never have to cry
> As long as there are shining
> Stars up in the sky

Dear Mr. Borman:

Although I have yet to thank you in person or letter, I want you to know that from the depths of my soul I want to thank you for giving me the opportunity to watch with my husband as our children grew up. One of my daughters is in the pharmacy field, and another has joined the Air Force. The paths they have chosen, I hope, will allow them to pay forward the generosity you have generously shared with my family. The twins, Dimitri and Hermione, are still in school, and I hope to attend their graduation in the future. I was but a child when you went to space, but the impact you had on my life will be what my family will remember most about you.

Love,
Zelphoe

Seventeen

Assassinations

When your focus is on saving your own life, it is easy to miss how your situation affects the people around you. If the situation is drastic enough, it can breed either friendship or enemies. In a 2014 conversation, E. Shirley Baca recalled her experience to a colleague, Robert, and me. She revealed several thorny situations she encountered because she stood in my corner. To recap briefly, Shirley started her push to remove Eric Serna as superintendent of insurance in 2004.

Shirley told us that she was at a "Welcome Event" in Mesilla for then-presidential candidate John Kerry, who was running against George W. Bush that year. Many Democratic elected officials were waiting in the home of former State Representative J. Paul Taylor. She was speaking to several New Mexico legislators she considered friends as they waited for Kerry to arrive. As the conversation turned to upcoming legislation, Shirley felt a cold hand press down on her exposed shoulder.

Governor Richardson had come up to her with a concerned look on his face and said, "I need to speak to you right now."

They went to a small room in a remote area of Representative Taylor's home. When they were in private, Governor Richardson cornered her. Towering over her, he poked her left shoulder, came down to her face, and said, "What the fuck do you think you are doing?"

Instinctively, Shirley pushed back and said, "I'm doing what the voters elected me to do, and what specifically are you referring to?"

Richardson responded, "This Maloney insurance investigation and insurance superintendent's office bullshit."

She retorted, "I was elected to uphold the public trust and do what's right, just as you were."

According to Shirley, the Governor pushed her aside and yelled, "You're just not a player!"

As he walked away, Shirley responded, "If being crooked means being a player, then no, I am not a player!"

I had no idea at the time, but this incident was a precursor to what I would later witness: the political assassination of Commissioner Shirley Baca at the hands of other Democrats at the time of my insurance denial.

A few weeks after her prickly encounter with Governor Richardson at the Kerry fundraiser, Shirley needed to take a plane from the Albuquerque airport for some PRC business. She was assigned a PRC motor pool car for the drive from Santa Fe to Albuquerque. That morning, she put her bags in the pool car and continued going about her duties the rest of the day. When she arrived at the airport, she checked her bags and proceeded to the gate. She heard a voice over the intercom asking her to go to a different gate. When she arrived there, not only were the police waiting in ambush to arrest her for possession of marijuana, but several news crews were set up to record the arrest.

According to news reports, fellow Democrats and PRC commissioners immediately turned their backs on Shirley. The following are excerpts from comments reported in the *Santa Fe New Mexican* shortly after her arrest:

> PRC Commissioner David King said he was stunned when told by the Associated Press that Baca had been arrested. "I know that she was one of the advocates to have a zero tolerance for drugs or alcohol" at the PRC, King said. She advocated immediate dismissal of any PRC employee when it comes to drugs or alcohol, he said.
>
> "We have a lot of sensitive positions here. We can't tolerate that (drugs and alcohol). I think that, as commissioners, we have to set a strong example," King said.
>
> Governor Bill Richardson said nobody is above the law.

Did someone plant marijuana in her suitcase while she was at the PRC building earlier that day? We have reason to believe they did. Other people had access to keys from the motor pool, and many had the motive to embarrass her. It is unlikely that news crews would be in place if the drugs were randomly found during the baggage scan. They were tipped off.

This was only the beginning. Shirley had a safe seat as a Democrat commissioner—that is unless another Democrat ran. The New Mexico Democratic Party, headed by the Governor, sponsored another candidate for her commission seat shortly after she got involved with my case. According to Shirley, the Democratic Party refused to fund her campaign, opting instead to fund another candidate. It turned into a three-person race, with two Democrat candidates and one Republican. The fix was in. Shirley didn't have a chance against the Governor-backed candidate. After decades of service as commissioner and in the legislature, her career was brought to an abrupt end in a few months. Our ally in the PRC was disgraced and discredited, ostensibly at the hands of Governor Bill Richardson.

Shirley was one of three persons stationed in the New Mexico PRC building to be removed for offering to help me. Joe Castellano, from the Office of Superintendent of Insurance, was another. In 2006, Governor Richardson appointed Morris Chavez as superintendent of insurance, and the PRC commissioners confirmed him. Robert and I were skeptical at first of another Richardson appointee. But Chavez and I shared a mutual friend in the Democratic Party. After he had firmly taken grasp of his position, negotiations began to trickle between us and the superintendent's office in late 2007.

At about the same time, *Bloomberg Markets* magazine had contacted Bill Webber about doing a national article about my case. Robert and I agreed to help. Chavez had agreed to interview for the article as well, although we were unaware of that at the time. The article "Toothless Watchdogs" was published in February 2008.

In late April 2010, after Robert had had a half dozen phone conversations with Chavez over those two years, a meeting at the superintendent's office was arranged among Chavez, Joel Newton, Robert, and me. It was uncomfortable walking into the office where Eric Serna had sat when he upheld the denial of my appeal. It became even more uncomfortable when the lawyer from the Office of General Council for the PRC, who had defended Serna, walked in to attend the meeting.

The short meeting drove me to a point. We wanted access to information Eric Serna had concealed so we could prove conspiracy between the then-superintendent of insurance and Lovelace to deny coverage to people with severe illness in exchange for monetary donations. Chavez agreed to conduct a full investigation and release any information he could to Joel. Robert and I were hopeful that we would finally get cooperation from the agency that had buried public information in an attempt to hide corruption.

Three things convinced us that Chavez was sincere. First, he projected a genuine nature—not arrogant—and he treated us with respect and apparent concern. Second was his cooperation with *Bloomberg Markets*. There was one line from the story that I appreciated most: "New Mexico Superintendent Morris Chavez wants to restore public confidence after others were accused of financial conflicts of interest and one regulator was convicted."

Third was the mutual friend who had known and worked with Chavez for decades.

Chavez's cooperation was big for us. Lovelace had managed to stall our case for more than five years, and new evidence confirming conspiracy would be detrimental to Lovelace. At last, we could move our case forward. A couple of weeks later, Robert received a personal call from Chavez. When Robert described the conversation to me, he looked disappointed and angry.

Chavez informed Robert that he was resigning as superintendent as of the close of business that day. He apologized that he would not be able to complete the investigation of Eric Serna, nor did he believe his replacement would continue the investigation. Chavez told Robert not to believe the impending news reports about the allegations a deputy superintendent made about sexual advances. He assured Robert he loved his wife and would never do such a thing. Chavez seemed truly distraught that his family would be impacted in a negative way. Then he wished us luck.

Lovelace had dodged another bullet.

All three people who offered to help us expose Eric Serna and Governor Richardson were eliminated from the PRC building within weeks of agreeing to help us. Doesn't that seem just a little too convenient?

Eighteen

Rebirth

After Frank Borman donated the money for my transplant, I was grateful and optimistic. But as Kim Young had warned me, there was a chance—relatively small as it was—that the procedure would not go as predicted and I would never see my children again.

Veronica was a mature seventeen-year-old high school senior whose circumstances had forced her to forfeit a great deal of her childhood. She never went to prom or graduation. Robert and I depended on her to handle things when I was sick. She helped with homework and even helped manage our business. She would grow up to be a woman with a constant nurturing spirit.

Otis was a fifteen-year-old, highly functioning autistic boy with the mental capacity of a six-year-old. He was bullied at school, and at times, it seemed there was little I could do about it. All he understood was that most of the time, Mom was not home, so he clung to Veronica. After Veronica left home, Otis clung to

Bridgette. He lives with us today but has strong connections with Bridgette and Veronica.

Bridgette was a ten-year-old who tried her best not to add to the complicated situation we were in. As a mature woman, she finally confessed that she was bullied at school by girls who pulled her hair, shoved her face in the sandbox, and made her eat sand. Later, boys tried to take advantage of her in sexual ways. She said she just dealt with it because she didn't want me to stress out over her situation. I wish I'd known so I could have tried to protect her. She grew up to be a strong woman with a no-nonsense attitude and a huge capacity for compassion. She was the first child born after I was diagnosed with lupus, but before I developed serious complications.

Our twins, Dimitri and Hermione, were four. They were the cutest children when they played off of each other to get what they wanted. It was amazing how one would distract us so the other could get things they shouldn't have, like fruit or cookies, from the table. They were a tag team and still are today.

The twins were a miracle. After a long discussion with my doctor late in 1999, Robert and I decided that having more children after Bridgette was not the best idea. I struggled with this because we wanted another child, but Robert took control and scheduled a vasectomy. Two days before his appointment, the doctor changed the HMO he serviced, and Robert had to reschedule with a new doctor. His next appointment was a month out. One week before his appointment, the doctor canceled, saying he had an emergency and would be out of town for a couple of weeks. Robert rescheduled for three weeks later. Robert received his vasectomy on schedule. Two weeks later, I found out I was pregnant. We were doubly surprised a few months later when we learned it was twins. It was a difficult pregnancy with plenty of complications, but looking back at August 2000, I wouldn't change a thing.

We needed to stay in Chicago for a month to prepare for the transplant, and then I could go home for a precious week before I returned for three to four months for the procedure. Although Frank Borman was paying for the transplant, Robert and I needed to raise $10,000 more to pay for travel and lodging. We sold everything we could, and Mike Gallagher, the journalist who had followed our story, let us place a fund request as part of the first story he wrote on the Eric Serna scandal. Fifty-five caring people gave donations ranging from five dollars to one hundred dollars. It looked tight, but we thought we could make it.

The Seneca Hotel in Chicago gave us a good rate for an extended stay. Mr. Foster, the long-term stay manager, was a saint and helped with all our accommodations, even supplying us with breakfast vouchers for the hotel cafe. The hotel was old and needed repairs, but the staff more than made up for the cosmetic shortfalls. Everyone—maids, doormen, front desk clerks—treated us with professionalism and dignity.

My mother stayed with the children. Robert was left with no choice but to entrust our sole source of income to three store managers he didn't know well our seventeen-year-old daughter, and his longtime accountant.

During my first two weeks in Chicago, I saw several specialists to verify that I was in good enough shape for the transplant. Every specialist had a similar question: "Why haven't your doctors treated you for this condition?" The heart specialist almost removed me from the program due to an enlarged heart. The gastrologist discovered colitis, the nephrologists worried about limited kidney function, and the pulmonologist found fibrosis and fluid in my lungs that needed to be removed. My body was on the verge of a total shutdown, and none of the records from Lovelace mentioned any of these complications.

I was placed on new medications, while others I had been taking were stopped or changed. Robert requested my medications at a nearby pharmacy that could deliver them. Lovelace rejected the request from out-of-network pharmacies to provide my medication. One of the drugs Dr. Oyama required me to change was my blood pressure medication. Three days later, Lovelace had not approved the request. I ran out of my old medication, and Lovelace would not authorize a refill of the current prescription or the filling of the new prescription.

On day four, I was unable to get out of bed on my own, and at ten o'clock in the morning, I heard Robert arguing on the phone with someone at Lovelace that my blood pressure was going out of control and I needed my prescription immediately. Robert told me that they said it would be approved. At eleven, Robert called the pharmacy, which informed us that it had not yet been approved. Robert tried again half an hour later and then again half an hour after that. I was screaming from pain, and it felt as if my eyes were going to burst out of my head. Robert called Kim Young, and she told him to bring me in immediately.

We caught a cab and rushed to Northwestern. We didn't have to check in and were taken to an exam room where Kim was ready. She checked my blood pressure, then ran and grabbed some blood pressure medication. Dr. Oyama met her in the room and told us he had ordered a hospital room for me, and he wanted me under observation until I could be stabilized. After two doses of medication spread thirty minutes apart, my blood pressure stabilized. I remained in the hospital for two days under constant observation.

I'm not sure what Kim said, but after she called Lovelace, the prescriptions were filled and delivered to my hotel that afternoon. In a subsequent conversation, Kim made light of Lovelace by saying, "They should be called Loveless rather than Lovelace."

After four exhausting weeks of examinations, interviews, and hospital stays, we were told that we needed to stay a few days longer for extra exams before I could travel home. Dr. Oyama told me he had never seen a candidate in as poor condition as I had been. After a few more days of testing, we got the green light to go home for a week. Then, we would need to return for the extraction of my "mother cells," the new cells generated in bone marrow, for the stem cell transplant.

The drama was over. I was going to spend time with my children. Robert and I boarded the plane to Denver, Colorado, where we would transfer planes to Albuquerque. As soon as we took off, I began having trouble breathing. By the time we landed in Denver, I thought I was going to die. Every breath sent a shooting pain across my back. Robert wanted to take me to the emergency room, but I refused. I just wanted to see my children. We boarded the plane, and it was all I could do to keep from screaming the entire flight.

When Veronica picked us up at the Albuquerque airport, Robert was pushing me in a wheelchair, and I was struggling for every breath. Robert immediately drove me to the Lovelace Women's Hospital. I was admitted and put on oxygen. It didn't seem fair. I had just left the hospital in Chicago, only to be thrust back into a hospital in Albuquerque before I could get home to see my children. My lungs were rapidly filling with fluid. The specialist came into the room and determined he needed to remove the fluid immediately. He asked me to sit in a chair and crouch over. I was no stranger to pain, but when the doctor pushed a needle through my back and into the lining of my lung to release the fluid, the pain was excruciating. The doctor removed about a liter of fluid that resembled pineapple juice. After the doctor drained my lungs, he asked me to cough. The room seemed to spin, and sharp pain shot across my back and chest with every breath.

After I was stable, Robert brought the children to see me. Bridgette had made me a cute card with a blue watercolor heart outlined in red. At the top, in large, bold green letters, she wrote, *I love my Mommy,* and at the bottom in blue were the words, *and Daddy.* Veronica, one of my little poets, also gave me a card splashed with color that read:

> I know her just as well as she knows me
> Staring into each other's eyes, searching deeply
> For the emotions that aren't spoken
> Nor shown in an admiration of a token
> I'm sorry you're not well on the day that lets me make up for my faults
> But you're busy fighting for your life and it halts
> Much appreciation that's due to you
> But I know you're strong and this won't conquer you
> Defeat I know you won't allow
> And you'll be coming home to be with your family
> But you're with us for a little while now

> You were the one that was always there for me when
> I needed it
> And I'm repaying because in this battle there is no
> talk of forfeit
> That's what your hope has taught me through the years
> Letting go and suppressing all fears
> And because of it I will never go down without a fight
> For standing up for what is right

I was in the hospital four of my seven days in Albuquerque. I was back home in bed the rest of the time, connected to an oxygen tank, with my head and shoulders propped up so I could breathe. The first three days in the hospital, the pulmonologist told me I might not be able to travel back to Chicago to finish my transplant. My desire to see my children had resulted in the possibility that the only treatment that could save my life might be an impossible three-hour flight away because of my diagnosis, pulmonary edema. I endured having the fluid drained from my lungs twice more.

On day four of my hospital stay, the pulmonologist walked in, holding a small stack of papers and wearing a smile. "I have your discharge papers," he said.

I immediately sat up, ignoring the pain. "You mean I can go to Chicago?"

The doctor stepped up next to the bed and said, "I think you'll be fine as long as you remain on oxygen. That means on the flight, as well as where you're staying."

I don't think I believed I was going back to Chicago until Robert wheeled me into our home later that day. Robert called the airline to make arrangements for oxygen. In a conversation Robert and I had after the transplant, he told me that the airline was very unreasonable, and the flight we were scheduled on had no available oxygen. They would not let him exchange or receive credit for the tickets because he had bought them at a special rate well in advance. They told him to buy new tickets on a different flight.

With only two days remaining before we needed to get back to Chicago, Robert was forced to get a title loan on our truck to afford the new tickets, which cost $1,200 one way because of the oxygen—which was provided for an additional $800. I was surprised that the airline would treat a terminally ill person in such a manner, but future interactions with this airline showed that this kind of treatment was par for the course. On the bright side, Dr. Oyama did not charge me for the extra treatments it took to prepare me for the transplant caused by the essential care Lovelace had failed to provide. Lovelace, to their credit, did have the oxygen machine the doctor ordered set up in my hotel room when I arrived.

When Robert and I returned to Northwestern, Dr. Oyama and Kim Young reevaluated me. My condition was borderline rejection, but he decided to continue. The next morning, I went to the harvesting center, the room where stem cells are harvested from the body. Kim connected me to what I can only describe as a modified dialysis machine. A tube was connected to a PICC line in my chest. A PICC line is a thin, soft, long catheter that is inserted into a vein. The tip is positioned in a large vein that carries blood into the heart. Blood was pumped into the machine for processing, then the blood was separated, and the unneeded portion was pumped back into my body.

During the several hours, while I was getting my mother cells harvested, Kim and Dr. Oyama stopped by frequently to talk to me and answer questions. Oddly, this was a fun experience because they and Robert lightened the mood with jokes. When I asked for some pictures, they smiled for the camera as they knelt close to me and gave me hugs. Robert noticed that jokes seemed to lighten my mood, so he bought me some joke books. He read me some of the jokes, but I rarely found them funny. Then Robert, the sweetheart that he is, astonished me by writing a joke book of his own. He called it *The Book of a Hundred Laughs*, and I got ten times that many laughs when he read it to me. He poked fun at the hospital by saying discounts might seem unnerving: "Vasectomies half off!" Satan did not want to be sued, so he had to place signs in hell that read, *Caution, Extremely Hot!*

In preparation for the chemotherapy, I followed Kim's advice, cut my hair off, and used a wig. The next several days of chemo resulted in my experiencing severe nausea, muscle pain, and devastating headaches. It did not, however, feel nearly as bad as the time it had been administered in Albuquerque. A nurse told me that some hospitals use a lower grade of Cytoxan for chemotherapy, which can cause more side effects. The lower-grade of product is cheaper and less pure.

That night, I wrote in my journal:

> Friday, May 20, 2005: Stem cell extraction is over. Just waiting for the white cell counts to go down and the side effects to come. I will be susceptible to infection and may need blood transfusion or even dialysis. I

don't know. My life is now in a waiting process, and patience and trust in God are all I have now.

After my white blood cell count diminished substantially, I was admitted into the hospital to continue my chemo and, hopefully, the introduction of a new immune system.

Living in a virtual bubble at Northwestern made me realize the severity of the situation. All staff and visitors had to go through an extensive decontamination process before they could enter the hospital wing, where I waited for the mother cells to reproduce. Robert was the only non-staff person allowed to visit me. He made sure he had no symptoms of illness, remained clean, and followed the strict rules for entering and leaving the secure hospital wing. That meant no outside food or drink and making sure only one of the several doors in and out of the wing was open at any given moment.

My white blood cell count was brought as close to zero as the doctors could bring it using chemotherapy. The staff on the hospital floor was extremely attentive and compassionate, but I lived in terror for days. Even a simple cold would have been life-threatening. I remember when Dr. Oyama, Kim Young, and Dr. Burt, the doctor who developed the procedure and had trained Oyama and Ann Traynor, walked into my hospital room when it was time to introduce my mother cells back into my body. Oyama held the syringe of stem cells that might give me a new life.

All three of them looked confident, not in a smug way but in a humble, enlightened manner. Robert asked one more time what we should expect. As Oyama prepared to inject the stem cells, Richard Burt explained that it usually took anywhere from four to ten days for the cells to react and begin production of the new immune system.

About an hour after the injection, there were no signs of any adverse reaction from the stem cells. Sporting a caring smile, Oyama told me to get some rest and that he would be back to check on me before he left the hospital for the day. That night, I wrote in my journal:

> The morning was nice. Later the blinds were open and the sky turned dark with bursts of lightning. It is frightening yet amazing from the twenty-fifth floor. I feel so lonely at times, but I know I have to do it for my family. I want to see my children grow. They are the most important things for me. In this world all I want is the best for them. I want them to have a mother, and I want to live for them. That is what gives me strength to go through all this, because it is not easy. By all means this is the hardest thing I have ever done in my entire life.

Behind the confident exterior Robert displayed in front of me most of the time, his true concern became evident when I overheard a phone conversation he had with Bob Mayfield almost two weeks after I completed the introduction of my stem cells at Northwestern. My eyes were closed, but I was not asleep.

"Hey, Bob. She's sleeping. It's already been longer than ten days, and her new immune system hasn't kicked in. I don't know what to tell the children when they ask me how she's doing."

Everyone was concerned that my white blood cells were not

increasing. It seemed my dream of a new life free of lupus was fading away.

On day eleven, in a last-ditch effort, Oyama ordered blood platelets to be introduced into my system. The next morning, he, Richard Burt, and Kim Young walked into my room, where Robert and I were discussing possible outcomes. Robert stood up; our full attention was on them. They were wearing huge smiles.

"Well, good morning!" Dr. Burt exclaimed.

Robert walked over and shook hands with the doctors. Kim stepped around and gave me a tearful hug. "Looks like somebody's growing," she said.

I cried with joy!

"It looks like adding platelets did it," Oyama announced.

Robert rushed over and gave me a gentle hug, and the doctors followed suit.

"You mean it worked?" I asked.

"Yep," Burt replied. "You can consider this your new birthday."

Robert squeezed my hand as tears filled his eyes.

Kim Young wiped her eyes: "This is the beginning of your new life."

Although my immune system was reproducing, my recovery was long and filled with a roller coaster of events. I was advised to keep several specialists informed of my condition after I returned to Albuquerque. Just before and during my transplant, my kidney function had been at borderline failure. Oyama told me there was a chance that the treatment could cause the remainder of my kidney function to diminish but that he had seen cases where the transplant actually regenerated kidney function.

It is a relief when wonderful news overshadows bad news. I was on my way home to be with my children. I was hopeful of a speedy recovery and a return to the role of functioning mother and wife. I would find out later, through a poem Bridgette wrote, how my absence affected my children.

Not Everyone Can
Mother please don't leave
I can't stand when you don't come back
No one likes to be deceived
Why not stay? Is it something I lack?
I can't stand when you don't come back
Running from your sickness but not far enough
Each time you return we get a knick-knack
I would rather have you than just useless stuff
Running from your sickness but not fast enough
Raising two kids and working so young
I would rather have you than just useless stuff
Tucking myself in with no songs to be sung
Raising 2 kids and working so young
No one likes to be deceived
Tucking myself in with no songs to be sung
Mother please don't leave

Nineteen

Another Deal with the Devil

Litigation reminds me of a game of truth or dare. One side demands something, and the other side determines if they should respond or dare the other side to prove the truth. Our experience was that mediation was no different.

We had been sitting in the small conference room at the Rodey Law Firm for what seemed like hours, waiting for a response to our offer to settle. Judge Garcia had ordered the mediation, but it was clear that Lovelace was just going through the motions with little sincerity or attention to the process.

I stood up and asked where the bathroom was. Robert walked with me. As we passed a large conference room, I stopped and pointed inside. Robert turned to look, and anger replaced frustration on his face. Franse and a group of individuals in well-tailored suits were sitting around a table, talking and laughing as they enjoyed fresh pastries and coffee.

It seemed obvious they had no intention of taking any offer we made seriously. The only reason they had invited us to the mediation was because Judge Garcia ordered it. The facts were on our side. We could prove corrupt behavior between Lovelace and the superintendent of insurance, but the judge would not allow the deposition of key witnesses. Without the testimony, we had no bargaining power to persuade Lovelace to entertain a settlement. We had to ask ourselves, "Why?"

As I noted earlier, attorney David Garza had suggested that we accept Judge Garcia over other possible judges. Garcia refused to rule on any motions to compel Lovelace or the superintendent of insurance to provide information or perform depositions. Every time we met in court, Nelson Franse maintained a smug attitude. The time clock in my life was no longer an issue, but it seemed what I considered the brick wall of corruption was still intact.

I was confused at a hearing Judge Garcia presided over on February 10, 2006. In an attempt to move the case forward, Bill Webber wanted to sidestep the insurance superintendent's objections to his involvement in the case so general discovery could resume. This is transcript from the February 10 hearing in Garcia's courtroom.

> THE COURT: I find that the issues with regard to due process, conflict of interest, those other issues, are being waived.
>
> MR. WEBBER: For the purposes of administrative appeal only.

> THE COURT: For purposes of the administrative appeal only. The only issue to be determined on the administrative appeal is whether or not the decision of the superintendent was correct and needs to be overturned.

Not once, but multiple times, Bill reminded the court that in no way was this request to relieve the common law and statutory claims of liability from Lovelace on the issue of conspiracy and corruption. Judge Garcia repeatedly asked Bill to consider the possible ramifications of his request. Garcia's comments made no sense to me, nor do I think they made sense to anyone else in the courtroom. Bill could not have been clearer about his intentions. Garcia's attitude was confusing because this hearing was a rehash of a hearing conducted on October 20, 2005. Joel would refer to this hearing in a motion filed with the court:

> The trial judge had actually already made a lengthy finding on the scope of the Maloneys' waiver in an order dated October 20, 2005, attached as Exhibit E. In the highlighted portions of that attached order, the trial judge literally "finds" that the Maloney "waiver" is strictly limited to the administrative appeal and solely for the purpose of expediting the coverage determination.

The power a judge has to dictate the flow of the courtroom had not been explained to me, but Judge Garcia left no doubt in my mind that this case was going nowhere. Over the next few hearings, Judge Garcia allowed for the depositions of several witnesses from our side but would not compel Lovelace to produce any relevant witnesses from their side for deposition. It was not until investigative reporter Mike Gallagher contacted Bill Webber about a story he was working on concerning my case that the question "Why?" was answered. Gallagher revealed that Judge Garcia's wife's law firm represented Eric Serna.

We went back to court on August 26, 2006. Joel and Bill were talking with us when the bailiff walked in and said, "All rise."

We stood up and waited for the judge to enter. This time, I had no hesitation about my ability to rise. As Judge Garcia walked in, I felt the tension thicken. He looked squarely at Joel and Bill, his gaze dark with anger. It was a short hearing focused on our motion for Judge Garcia to recuse himself. Bill outlined several reasons why he should do so:

> Plaintiffs made it clear that the appearance of impropriety encompasses more than just the fact the judge's wife's law firm actively represented Eric Serna. We raised the issue of the "nexus" between other Con Alma contributors and the judge's wife... We spoke to the fact that there were an unknown number of witnesses that would come up in this case who were Con Alma contributors and whose connections to Judge Garcia's wife raise concern. For instance, it now appears that Judge Garcia's wife sits on the advisory board of Century Bank, which along with Lovelace, is one of Con Alma's biggest

contributors . . . Guy Riordan, who handled Con Alma investments, was a substantial contributor to a political campaign treasured by Judge Garcia's wife. But Guy Riordan wasn't the only contributor:

Nestor Romero, Eric Serna's auditor, who was assigned to audit Lovelace.

Robert Desiderio, Executive Director of Con Alma.

Quinn Lopez, Superintendent Serna's legal counsel who was directly involved in the Maloney appeal.

Rio Chama Restaurant, owned by Gerald Peters, who is also the largest owner of Century Bank.

The nexus would not be so troubling if this was a dog bite case. But this is a political corruption case, and Lovelace proposed findings to remove the heart of the issue.

Nelson Franse was not about to let "his" judge walk away without a fight. "If a judge under rules should keep the case," he argued, "he's required to keep the case, and so we are going to be looking at our options to have this reviewed by some other court, to, in our view, confirm your thinking that there is no reason for you to get off the case."

Bill Webber and Nelson Franse went round about again, and then, without warning, Judge Garcia said in an irritated voice,

"At this point, I am going to assume I am off the case." Garcia defended his position that he should not recuse himself in the Order on Plaintiff's Motion to Disqualify, stating, "I was unaware of the representation of Mr. Serna in connection with these matters by my wife's firm until late 2006, when the matter was brought to my attention by a journalist." As a single woman, I might have bought that excuse, but as a married woman, not a chance.

This news was devastating, not only from a legal perspective, but from a humanitarian perspective as well. The only bright spot was that we were at last free from under the oppressive thumb of Judge Garcia, who had wasted over two years of time and resources and ultimately would have sealed my death had Frank Borman not interceded.

There are times when a person suspects foul play, and there are times when it's shoved in your face. Judge Timothy Garcia recused himself based on a conflict of interest, but only after stalling our lawsuit for several years. If not for the diligent investigation of Mike Gallagher, my case might have been stalled indefinitely. This lost time could not be recovered, and the delay created additional financial hardship for our family, as well as one of the attorneys fighting for us.

Robert had refinanced our home at less than reasonable terms and fell behind on tax payments, and all the while, Lovelace kept increasing our premiums and co-payments. One of our attorneys was struggling to make ends meet as well. Lovelace and their attorneys remained fully funded and took every opportunity to prolong the lawsuit.

It was over four months since Judge Garcia had recused himself on August 6, 2006. We had not yet been appointed a new judge, but Robert and I were hopeful that a new judge would move our case along and stop the stonewalling from the superintendent of insurance and Lovelace. Robert went out and retrieved the mail. Inside, among all the past-due notices, was a copy of an order written by Garcia.

When Robert walked inside, I knew something was wrong. He didn't say a word to me. He walked past me in a daze and continued into his office, where he called Joel. I followed him in and heard him ask, "Can he do that? Can he make that ruling four months after he has officially recused himself?"

Garcia had written an order on our case four months after he recused himself.

I saw the helplessness in Robert's eyes and understood why when he told me Joel's response: "I have never seen such an unethical action committed by a judge. He has gone years without making a ruling on any substantial hearings or motions, dragging his feet at every turn. And now he basically throws out half our case after he has officially recused himself."

Joel summed it up in the appeal he filed with the New Mexico Supreme Court:

> The parties agreed to a form of order identical in all respects, with one major exception: Finding No. 6 of Lovelace's proposed order. Lovelace sought a substantive finding not discussed at the August 26, 2006 hearing, a finding the judge had specifically declined to make in an earlier hearing held February 14, 2006. This new finding was made almost four months after the judge announced he was "off the

case." The scope of the finding in that written order of disqualification effectively dismisses common law and statutory claims against Lovelace for insurance bad faith under the guise of voluntary waiver by the Maloneys in the administrative appeal phase of the case... In his disqualification order, for the first time, the former trial judge found that the waiver made solely in the context of the administrative appeal "would encompass... any allegations... (the Maloneys) might seek to pursue in the context of common law or statutory claims . . ." Thus, after recusing himself he effectively dismissed common law and statutory claims of the Maloneys against Lovelace.

The portion of my lawsuit that contained the lack of due process by Eric Serna, based on bribes, would never be explored. Serna would not have to testify, nor could we use the insurance company's bribes to Con Alma as part of the case against Lovelace. The public would never get the full story of how the New Mexico government and insurance companies conspired to disenfranchise the citizens of New Mexico.

Joe Castellano had given me a list of more than thirty people Lovelace had denied for similar causes but did not have the resources to fight back. Ultimately, Joe Castellano was fired from the Office of Superintendent of Insurance after denying an offer from Serna for a promotion and releasing documents to our attorneys.

A few weeks after Garcia's order of recusal was submitted and half our case wiped out, Governor Richardson appointed

Judge Garcia to the New Mexico Court of Appeals—a big promotion and what looked like a payoff for his unfavorable treatment of Robert and me.

Our children didn't care about the litigation. They just understood that Mom was home again.

Twenty

Firestorm

The conspiracy between the superintendent of insurance and New Mexico insurance companies could continue uninterrupted because of Judge Garcia's ruling. Judge Garcia had let the politicians off the hook. But for the sake of families like ours, we had to continue the fight we began in 2004.

Our case was setting precedents. It had begun with the investigation Robert and I started, which led to Mike Gallagher's revealing articles. Ultimately, it developed into a joint investigation by the FBI and the New Mexico attorney general's office into the PRC, the superintendent of insurance, and the governor's office. Our attorneys had released all the information they had on Eric Serna to the United States prosecutor.

Because of the media exposure, New Mexico state senator Mary Kay Papen introduced legislation that would take the final appeal before litigation from the appointed superintendent of insurance and place it in the hands of the elected PRC commissioners. Robert and I supported this move and drove to Santa Fe on February 17, 2005, for a discussion of this matter and to request the PRC support the legislation.

Senator Papen and several other prominent officials from both political parties pushed for the changes that Papen's bill demanded. Robert and I spent several days pleading with state legislators to support the bill. In the end, everyone's hard work paid off. The bill passed unanimously in the New Mexico House of Representatives and moved to the Senate. After a full debate, the bill was passed with only a single "no" vote.

We had accomplished the impossible. We had unified New Mexico, and the tyranny of the superintendent of insurance would soon come to an end. The only obstacle was Governor Bill Richardson. No one we talked to in the legislature believed Richardson would risk political clout by vetoing a bill with such media coverage and almost unanimous support of the legislature.

But he did.

In an interview with Mike Gallagher, published in the newspaper on July 2, 2006, Senator Papen was quoted as saying, "I was never told why it was vetoed . . . I assumed the governor was looking out for Eric." The response from the governor's office, reported in the same story, was that "the bill was vetoed because of technical problems."

On another trip Robert and I took to speak with then-PRC chair Ben Ray Lujan Jr., we again were hopeful. When the doors of the elevator opened on the second floor of the PRC building, we witnessed a madhouse. Federal officials armed with dollies were wheeling stacks of file boxes out of the superintendent's office. Several news reporters watched, shouting questions and taking photos of the FBI raid. Robert and I walked toward the PRC hearing room. At that moment Eric Serna dashed out of the hearing room and continued past us toward his office. His face was covered as he held his coat up over his head. Robert shook his finger and shouted out at Serna, "You can run, but you can't hide."

An insider at the Office of Superintendent of Insurance confirmed to me that the day before the raid, under Serna's direction, department employees had shredded documents until the wee hours of the morning.

A few days after the raid, Robert and I were sitting in a hotel lobby waiting for our attorneys. They had scheduled for us to have lunch and discuss our case. As they approached, we overheard Bob say, "I had breakfast with Gallagher this morning to further discuss the information you found out about Bill Madison being shaken down by Joe Ruiz and Eric Serna."

Joel responded, "What did he think about that?"

"He fed that information to the FBI. Ruiz is about to be indicted. If he turns on Serna, the whole Con Alma mess will come into play. We can get Serna's testimony from the federal prosecutor."

We never got to use any of the testimony from this investigation, but Serna was forced to retire as superintendent of insurance on June 14, 2006. Prior to his retirement, he was suspended with full pay and benefits for over a month, and by staying on until June 14, he qualified for a full pension package. The PRC could have forced him out sooner but opted to let Serna qualify for all benefits. Joe Ruiz was indicted on thirty-one counts on August 24, 2007, and, according to several news reports, the FBI was investigating Governor Richardson's involvement in several "Pay to Play" scandals.

With increasing media coverage and indictments in the wind, Robert and I were optimistic that the dealings at the PRC would finally be examined. He had tried to obtain information from the Office of the Superintendent of Insurance on several previous occasions while investigating the insurance company's profit margins. In New Mexico, insurance premiums are set by a flat-rate profit margin. That is, a company is allowed to profit from providing insurance at a pre-determined margin. The total dollar amount it costs to provide care, plus the profit margin, is used to determine policy premiums. The issue is not whether the concept is fundamentally fair or unfair. It's a matter of how it's implemented. An insurance company is allowed to estimate costs for the next year and then estimate the premiums required. Robert reasoned that at least one time, Lovelace had to have overestimated the cost and, in turn, should have issued a refund for the overpayment. We never received a refund.

Robert went to the PRC to retrieve what should have been public records on the PRC's review of Lovelace's estimates for determining premiums. The person who had the files was indignant and refused to let Robert look at them. Robert shot back, "What if a PRC commissioner wants to look at them?"

The irate man shouted back, "No one can look at them."

In other words, apparently, "no one" was in a position to verify Lovelace's estimates of cost for insurance premiums.

Twenty-One

A Perfect Match

Dr. Burt had two concerns when I left Chicago—my heart and kidneys—and gave me orders to have doctors in Albuquerque monitor their function. My cardiologist had seen me briefly a few weeks prior to the stem cell transplant. At that brief encounter, I noticed his expression, which reminded me of what I saw on many other faces at that time. It was an empathetic look, as though they were thinking, this might be the last time I see this person.

The first time he saw me after my stem cell transplant, the cardiologist did a double take when he entered the exam room. "You're here!" he exclaimed as he walked over to the desk.

"What do you mean?" I asked.

"You were so sick," he replied as he adjusted his computer screen. "It's just good to see you." He looked over the test results of the past year and then asked me to sit on the exam table. "This is remarkable. The enlarged heart is gone—back to normal."

"I thought you told us it would never return to normal."

"I've never seen anything like this," he said with amazement. "It must be from the stem cell transplant."

I would later discover through another cardiologist that this doctor had never told me the whole story about my condition. I had had a heart attack before my transplant, and we were never told about it.

Although the news about my heart was exciting, other health issues persisted. When you're strapped into the dialysis seat, surrounded by other patients who have lost hope of a transplant, you just want to cry as you imagine what your future may hold. Suddenly, your anger about who is responsible for your condition fades into the question, *How do I get out of here?* But when the opportunity to escape the bondage of dialysis occurs, it comes with a hefty price—a deep sense of guilt.

After the successful stem cell transplant, my lupus symptoms faded away. My ability to breathe without oxygen returned. My blood pressure stabilized, I could eat normally, and I regained weight. All aspects of my life improved dramatically, except for my kidney function.

Robert and I resisted my renal doctor's recommendation to begin dialysis in June 2005. In fact, he was angry that I had not started dialysis immediately after returning from Chicago. We were hopeful that, like the dramatic improvement in my lungs, intestines, stomach, and heart, my kidneys would improve over time. As a precaution, I registered with the Mayo Clinic in Scottsdale, Arizona, and actively tested myself to be a transplant candidate. Family members who wanted to be donors were evaluated, but none qualified.

After a few fretful weeks, we reluctantly accepted the fact that dialysis would need to be part of my life. Since my kidneys couldn't do their job anymore, we needed dialysis to help remove waste, salt, and extra water from my body so they wouldn't build up, as well as help control my blood pressure and maintain a safe level of certain chemicals in the bloodstream.

It would require a half day, three times a week. I was hopeful dialysis would be short term. Dr. Burt believed, based on other patient outcomes, that the stem cell transplant I had received could still improve my kidney function in the near future.

Dialysis is a horrible miracle of modern medicine. I experienced severe muscle cramps, high blood pressure, fatigue, and unstoppable headaches. My whole life revolved around my next dialysis session. The first time I walked into a dialysis clinic, it reminded me of walking into a cemetery. Dialysis machines lined the walls, reminiscent of a row of tombstones. Next to each machine sat a reclining chair, like a casket waiting for a body to be placed in it. The patients who occupied the chairs reminded me of the zombies from the movie *Night of the Living Dead*. The best phrase I can think of to describe it is, "Gloom abounds!"

Managing blood pressure is a top priority for dialysis patients and a difficult task for doctors. It was common for my doctor to change my blood pressure medication or change the dose of a current medication. On one occasion, my blood pressure kept spiking over several days. In an attempt to control it, the dialysis doctor prescribed clonidine, a drug that can relieve high blood pressure quickly. I took the dose that night when my blood pressure spiked. The next morning, I felt weak and drowsy. When I went in for dialysis, the technician took my blood pressure. Without a word, she ran off and returned with the doctor. His face turned white. He immediately ordered a saline drip. I later discovered that my blood pressure had dropped so dangerously low that my organs weren't getting the blood flow they needed to sustain life.

One of the most difficult aspects of dialysis is coping with the loss of fellow patients. One day, the person who usually sits next to you doesn't show up. Some of these patients have been waiting for a transplant for several years. Some had simply opted to discontinue dialysis, even if that meant they would die in a matter of days. Other patients were hospitalized but returned after a few weeks. Some of them were having limbs amputated because chronic kidney disease patients have a relatively high risk of developing peripheral artery disease. They have reduced blood flow to the lower extremities, and can lose a foot or leg because of it.

Blood work is drawn at every dialysis session. The information is used to monitor filter requirements. Twenty-one days after I started dialysis, my blood work showed improved kidney function, just as Dr. Burt had predicted. It seemed that my kidney function had rebounded to an acceptable level, and I was taken off dialysis.

I felt as though I were dreaming. Robert took me home, and a few friends showed up later for a small celebration.

Two days later, I started becoming increasingly fatigued. By day seven, my kidney function had declined back to where it was before I was released from dialysis. The stem cell transplant did have a positive effect, but the damage done during my IVIG treatment was too severe, and the stem cell transplant could not rectify it. I was, therefore, returned to the bondage of dialysis, my pardon revoked by the severity of the damage.

At one session in February 2006, I sat in my chair as warm blood drained from my arm into the dialysis pump to be filtered before being returned cool into my body. I was watching the news on one of the televisions placed around the facility when a woman across from me went into rapid convulsions, then suddenly stopped and lay limp in her dialysis chair. Several of us yelled for help as we were unable to move from our seats. One by one, the entire staff rushed over to help her as the rest of us sat helpless. One staff checked for a pulse, while another ran to the phone at the end of the hall and others prepared to stop treatment and remove the lines from her arms. In the distance, I heard sirens, and by the time she was disconnected, EMTs rushed and took her away. She never returned.

During the yearlong torture of my time on dialysis, I desired nothing more than to escape. My doctor placed me on the transplant list, but my chances of receiving a transplant were slim.

In an attempt to lighten the mood, I would try to joke with the dialysis technicians. During one session, the technicians were watching a football game. They asked, "Do you like football?"

"No," I said. "Look at those guys. They're wearing tight pants. I watch soccer." We all had a little laugh.

Robert usually sat next to me while I received dialysis, but on October 6, 2006, he returned home to check on the twins. I sat alone, tethered to a tube filled with my circulating blood. Technicians walked about, checking dialysis machines that would beep every so often if they needed adjusting. As I watched the revolving door of dialysis patients, I wondered what would happen to my family and me. I noticed that a person receiving a transplant was very rare. In fact, I couldn't remember anyone who had left because they received a transplant. The loss of hope forced its way into my thoughts as sadness filled my heart. It often occurred to me that I would not survive for very long, and I wondered what would become of my children if I was not around.

I was wondering what my children were doing when my phone rang. I answered it and heard an unfamiliar voice.

"This is Mary at the Mayo Clinic in Scottsdale, Arizona. Is this Mrs. Maloney?"

"Yes."

"I have wonderful news," she said as I transitioned my thoughts from my children to the soft-spoken person on the line. "We have a kidney with a six-point out of a six-point match for you."

I sat for a beat, trying to grasp what she had just said. "I'm not up to talking right now," I said. "Can you please call my husband?"

After a moment of awkward silence, she responded that she would, but she needed to talk to him right away. I gave her Robert's number, which she said she already had. I didn't think about it at the time, but she probably thought I was rude. The fact is, I was in a state of disbelief and denial, so much so that I felt sick to my stomach.

Thirty minutes later, the slow-motion world of dialysis picked up to a frenzy. Robert didn't realize that the woman from the Mayo Clinic hadn't had the opportunity to tell me why she was calling. My technician came walking toward me with an enormous smile. Just then, Robert called. "Hey, honey. Do they have you off the dialysis machine yet?"

Puzzled, I replied, "You know I won't be finished for half an hour."

"No. They're supposed to take you off now. Our flight leaves in about an hour and a half. I already packed our things and will be there in ten minutes to pick you up. Go ahead and finish, but we'll have to hurry from there."

As I hung up the phone, stunned, a grinning technician walked up and said, "I'm so happy for you," as she prepared to take me off the dialysis machine. The whole room was spinning as it sank in that the Mayo Clinic had a kidney for me!

As our plane touched down in Phoenix, Robert called the clinic to let them know we had arrived. The person on the other end of the line told Robert that the timing was perfect and the kidney would be arriving on another flight in a few minutes.

The two weeks of testing we'd done at the Mayo Clinic in the summer of 2006 had paid off. Robert and I had asked many questions and thought we had a good understanding of what receiving a kidney would require. We were anticipating a six-year wait to move to the top of the donor list. What we didn't know was that the Mayo Clinic looks at six antigens when determining a suitable donor. One nurse told me that a three-antigen match is the minimum allowed. The higher the antigen match, the greater the probability of a successful transplant.

Here is what this all means: Antigens are markers on the body's cells that help your body differentiate between self and non-self. The body relies on this to protect itself by recognizing and attacking something foreign, like bacteria or viruses. My body was less likely to send white blood cells to attack a transplanted organ if the antigens matched.

There are lots of different antigens, but six have been identified as having an important role in transplantation: A, B, and DR antigens. There are two antigens for each letter. Parents pass these antigens down—three (A, B, and DR) from the mother and three (A, B, and DR) from the father. Children born to the same parents may inherit the same combination or a different combination of antigens. In other words, you have a reasonably good chance of having siblings with a match.

But except for identical twins and some brothers and sisters, it is very rare to get an exact match between two people. The chance of finding an exact match with an unrelated donor is about one in 100,000.

When we arrived at the Mayo Clinic, I was rushed through admitting and taken to a room. The nurse who was to prepare me for the surgery walked in and began explaining the procedure. At some point, she referred to the fact that the kidney had a six-antigen match. Robert said that was great, and I said something to the effect of, "That's nice."

The nurse looked at me with an unbelieving stare. "You don't understand. You have a perfect match. I have never seen this before. In fact, no one here has ever seen this before. It's like winning the lottery!"

Then I understood: the reason I had been bumped up five years on the waiting list was because of the rare occurrence of a perfect-match kidney.

Over the next several hours, the staff did blood work and monitoring. Robert sat by my side off and on, unsuccessfully trying to hide his anxiety. The tension broke when the nurse came in and announced, "We still need to see if there is any reaction from your antibodies to the kidney. We should get the results shortly." My blood had been tested almost twenty times before for possible live donor transplants, and in every instance, my body had rejected them. At the moment the nurse mentioned testing my blood, every encounter crashed in on me in a moment of utter panic.

Instinctively, I asked, "What happens if there's a reaction?"

"Then we go to patient number two."

Robert stood up. "You mean you have another person waiting for this kidney?"

Her smile quickly changed. "Yes. But don't worry! Your wife is a perfect match. Worst case scenario, patient two is already here at the hospital." She fidgeted. "I probably shouldn't have told you that."

Here I was, waiting to see if my body wouldn't reject the donor kidney, while the person I had skipped over was just two doors down, wondering who knows what. I will be brutally honest: I wanted that kidney. I felt deeply for the woman down the hall, and I wish the nurse hadn't told me she was there. In the end, I rationalized that I had done nothing wrong to jump the line. I could not control my antigens.

This situation seemed cruel. I didn't realize doctors had to make these types of choices. At the decision of the doctor, one of us was going home empty-handed. I began to breathe deeply and decided to calm down and try to fall asleep so I didn't have to contemplate this dilemma. Looking back, this seems weird, but at the time, it made perfect sense. Soon, I cleared my mind and fell asleep.

Moments later, the nurse walked in and said with a smile, "There is zero rejection. The kidney is yours."

Twenty-Two

Scapegoating

Sacrifice is expected in politics, albeit in different forms. Sometimes, it takes the form of a scapegoat. In the Bible, this literally refers to a goat set loose in the wilderness after a high priest symbolically lays the sins of his people on the animal's head. In politics, scapegoats are selected by those in power to hide embarrassing errors or crimes.

Eric Serna, who had Joe Ruiz to carry his sins, is the President, General Counsel/lobbyist with Goldwater Taplin Group. The Goldwater Taplin Group was founded in Florida in 2006, the same year Eric Sena was forced to resign as the New Mexico Superintendent of Insurance. He now assists the insurance industry in finding solutions to regulatory issues.

Bill Richardson, who ran for president of the United States in 2008, had any number of scapegoats, some of whom were named in earlier chapters. They apparently weren't strong enough to carry his sins into the wilderness, however, since he was forced to withdraw as President Barack Obama's Commerce Secretary nominee because of a federal grand jury investigation into pay-to-play charges. Oh, and that just might have had something to do with Robert and me.

Scapegoats sometimes meet a justice-hungry public's need to punish someone for wrongdoing; the real culprit gets away because the itch has been scratched. When a person realizes he's being sacrificed, he sometimes is willing to divulge what he knows about the real criminal—but it's often too late at that point. Scapegoats generally don't find the media receptive to their story, ostensibly fueled and tainted by the desire for revenge.

Robert and I read about the verdict in the Joe Ruiz case in the newspaper. When we discussed it with our lawyers, we discovered that one of them was at the court when the verdict was read.

On January 28, 2008, Ruiz sat as the jury walked in, ready to announce their findings on the thirty-one indictments. His counsel, Tim Padilla, and co-counsel, Tom Tabet, sat by his side. Padilla stared at the floor as Tabet stared at the jury box. Judge Bill F. Johnson waited for the jurors to take their seats, ignoring Ruiz. Only a handful of people, including members of the press, were in the courtroom. The bailiff stood close to the judge. After the last juror sat down, Judge Johnson asked, "Jury, have you reached a verdict?"

The jury foreman stood. "Yes, your honor. We have reached a unanimous decision on all thirty-one counts."

Judge Johnson ordered the bailiff to bring him the verdict from the foreman. The bailiff took the verdict and handed it to the judge. The judge looked it over for a moment before returning it to the bailiff, who took it back to the jury foreman.

The judge told Ruiz to rise for the reading of the verdict. Ruiz and his lawyers rose. The judge cleared his throat and asked, "On the first indictment of conspiracy to commit extortion, what is your verdict?"

The foreman replied, "Not guilty, your honor."

All mumbling stopped, and Ruiz's frown began to resemble a slight smile.

"On the second indictment of extortion, what is your verdict?" the judge asked.

The foreman took a deep breath and said, "On this and the remaining indictments, we find the defendant guilty."

There was a quiet roar of comments among the observers. Ruiz dabbed his eyes, then covered them with a handkerchief. He was flushed and reached down to the table to steady himself as his lawyers helped him sit down.

Ruiz looked up at Padilla and mumbled something like, "You told me it was all handled."

The judge brought down his gavel. "Order in the courtroom." As the commotion silenced, he said, "I'm sorry, Mr. Foreman, but you will need to read each count out loud. Please rise, Mr. Ruiz."

After the verdict, Ruiz was escorted down the steps in handcuffs. Reporters clamored for a statement. Ruiz stopped and said, "Wait! Wait a moment." Most people hushed to listen. Scott Sandlin reported Joe Ruiz's response in an article that appeared in the *Albuquerque Journal* on July 16, 2008: "I'm sorry . . . for many things. I'm sorry I ever met Eric Serna. I'm sorry I took his offer of employment. I'm sorry I took his word that everything I did was legal." Ruiz lowered his head as officers escorted him to a white van. Reporters erupted into a frenzy and followed him to the van.

According to Joe Castellano, Ruiz had accepted the advice of Eric Serna to use Democratic Party attorneys. In later discussions with the press, he admitted that he was under direct orders from Serna when it came to extorting money from insurance providers, but that window was closed. Now, all his words were tainted outbursts from a felon. Serna, on the other hand, walked away from this crime a free man.

Ruiz went to federal prison for four years while Serna continued his professional career in the private sector, supplemented by a full pension from the state of New Mexico. Once again, a powerful man escaped with little more than a bruised public opinion. How many times, in other states or other countries, does the story repeat itself?

Twenty-Three

New Hope

By the end of 2008, Robert and I had shifted focus in regard to Lovelace. I was now on Medicare and no longer relied on the company for my medical needs. Robert was in the process of trying to sell our business before we were forced to close the shops. My lupus was in full remission, and my kidney transplant was about to enter a third year with zero rejection. After years of fighting with Lovelace and discovering their business practices, the lawsuit transformed into a fight for justice rather than a fight for life. Lovelace had been able to hide unnerving details about its operations. Robert and I were determined to expose them so the insured could be informed about red flags when they were denied coverage.

A new judge was a welcome change to a stalled lawsuit. It was January of 2009 when we first encountered Judge Daniel Sanchez. Fear mixed with optimism as we drove to Santa Fe for our first hearing with the new, unknown judge. As we sat and watched the short, bearded man wearing a robe interact with the lawyers in the room, I became calm. Judge Sanchez came across as a decent person who was legitimately trying to bring himself up to speed on my case. Robert held my hand tightly as the hearing came to a close and we waited to hear the judge's response to Joel Newton.

After a tense silence, Judge Sanchez said, "I see. Okay. Very well. If there is nothing else on this particular issue, we'll be adjourned."

The court reporter stopped typing. Joel spoke up. "Your Honor, just looking forward, we have a June trial date, and we've got a number of discovery motions and a motion to amend the complaint that has been pending since January of '06."

My nervousness was subsiding, but it seemed Robert was still anxious as he leaned forward in anticipation of the judge's response.

In a stern tone, Judge Sanchez said, "It's been five years, and Lovelace has failed to respond to plaintiff's requests for depositions and documents. I'm retiring in May of next year, and I assure you this case will finish before I do. We will set up for jury selection in December—and I'd better see significant progress in the meantime."

Finally, after years of suppression at the hands of Judge Garcia, it appeared we were getting closer to unveiling the truth about Lovelace's business practices. But Lovelace continued the stalling game. Defendants refused to supply documents or schedule relevant depositions. The June trial date was lost.

At the next hearing on June 29, 2009, Judge Sanchez heard

objections from Lovelace as to why it did not need to supply documents or complete depositions. He responded, "With respect to Request for Production No. 3, manuals, internal procedures re: Mrs. Maloney's claims, the objection is overruled. Those will be produced, and they will be produced for a time period from 2003 through 2006."

Bill and Joel seemed hopeful we could proceed on a level playing field under Sanchez. Bob Mayfield was not at this hearing. His health had deteriorated, and the five-hour drive from Las Cruces was too much for him to endure. Although his physical health had waned, he remained sharp when it came to legal strategy, and he attended telephonically.

Over the next several months, Bill and Joel traveled to several states, from California to Massachusetts, conducting depositions. A jury selection service had been contacted to aid in our jury selection. Joel spent hours a day reviewing the facts of the case so he could discuss strategy with Bob and Bill. This was a time of momentum, and our legal team was determined to complete as much of the necessary work that would be needed for Judge Sanchez to schedule a trial date.

Several hearings were held before the one we were looking forward to in December 2009. Nelson Franse resisted as much as he thought he could get away with, rescheduling depositions as often as possible in order to frustrate Joel and Bill and to get Robert and me to give up the lawsuit. In a Status Report filed with the court, Bill Webber wrote:

> Plaintiffs sent Lovelace council a letter over a week ago, which summarizes much of this Status Report

and invites Lovelace to complete compliance with this Court's Order. That invitation has been declined. Instead, Lovelace asked us to cancel corporate depositions going to this very issue because the noticed depositions did not comply with the letter of the law on notice. We did so. And so the spirit of the Court's direction is sacrificed and the discovery that could have finalized our evaluation reported is again put off until after the December 7, 2009 Status Conference.

A few months earlier, Joel had written this to the court:

In June, I set the depositions of major witnesses for two weeks in July 2009, only to have Lovelace say that only two of the twelve deponents could be available. Lovelace then agreed to provide dates and work corporately to schedule the depositions in August. You agreed to schedule these depositions prior to the mediation.

Lovelace's actions in 2009 were part of a long string of similar behavior stemming back to 2004. In the same motion mentioned above, it states, "This Court has had to vacate scheduling orders, with trial dates, six times. This would be the seventh."

Franse also enlisted the help of a young lawyer, Brian Brack, and brought him to one of Judge Sanchez's hearings. The judge seemed distracted by his presence. Sanchez's face turned red on a couple of occasions when the young attorney addressed him.

The fact was that the young lawyer was the nephew of a powerful federal judge. Was he brought in to display the power and influence of the Rodey Law Firm? This was another time when I went through the stages of grief quickly: I first denied that this could happen, was angry that it might be, wanted to find out what our bargaining chips were, and felt depressed that we had an unscrupulous assault once again—but then, as with my medical situation, neither I nor Robert ever got to the acceptance stage. No!

In the end, Joel had the advantage. He had studied this case for years, from top to bottom. I believe he knew more about Lovelace than any single person at Lovelace did. Franse, on the other hand, had not taken the case seriously. In fact, under Judge Garcia, he'd had no reason to take the case seriously. For Franse, it was time to play catch-up, and Judge Sanchez was not about to go into overtime. He was scheduled to retire.

Although Franse was playing hardball, the Albuquerque Chamber of Commerce, from whom we had purchased our Lovelace plan, was cooperative. The mission of a Chamber of Commerce is to unify merchants for the purpose of promoting local business events and to represent local businesses on business-related issues such as health care. The Chamber turned over what they described as all relevant documents they could find regarding Lovelace and the Chamber. After reviewing the documents and conducting an initial deposition of Andrea Nash on September 16, 2009, Joel outlined his discoveries beautifully in a Motion for Sanctions filed with the court:

> This court ordered Lovelace to produce the health services agreement in effect in 2004 between the

Albuquerque Chamber of Commerce and Lovelace. In response, Lovelace produced a document, unsigned by the Chamber, ever. The Plaintiffs took deposition of the Chamber representative, who denies that the Chamber even has the contract document Lovelace tendered as "the agreement." In fact, the only contract the Chamber had with Lovelace was dated December 7, 2004, and it is a completely different document than the "Health Services Agreement."

The December 2004 contract is called a "Broker Agreement," a contract created after this litigation began. It is a document created because for years Lovelace had been paying the Chamber a 2.5 % commission on premiums, a kickback of sorts of a portion of Chamber members' insurance premiums paid to Lovelace . . . When this litigation began, apparently Lovelace and the Chamber needed a contract in place to try and explain the commission.

Lovelace's Handbook says, "The premiums for these benefits have been based on service being provided by Plan Providers." Nowhere did Lovelace disclose that the premiums are also based on an undisclosed kickback and/or illegal rebate to the Chamber, a group which had already charged the Maloneys a membership fee for the privilege of purchasing the Group policy from Lovelace.

In short, there is no contract for health services with the Chamber, and Lovelace has hidden that fact. Lovelace had plenty of motive to pass the unsigned document off as such a contract. Its biggest hurdle in hiding its problem of "no contract" is that the Chamber has never seen the document, much less signed it. The Chamber only has a contract, which tries to remedy violation of State Law with the Department of Insurance for Lovelace's undisclosed payment of, what Plaintiffs believe, are illegal commissions and rebates. Lovelace seems to think its duty is to the Department of Insurance, because it never tried to remedy the real problem of failing to disclose to its members its various contract (or actually, no contract) problems.

In other words, Lovelace proffered a document which it knew was never signed by the Chamber, that the Chamber did not agree to or even have in its position at anytime material relevant to this lawsuit—or even presently—pass off as "the contract."

On November 11, 2009, Joel deposed Andrea Nash of the Albuquerque Chamber of Commerce a second time about the Chamber's role as an insurance broker for Lovelace. Cole was a well-dressed woman who looked stressed or even frightened as she sat waiting for Joel to begin. Her legal counsel sat next to her.

Right off the bat, Joel asked, "So you have brought in over eight hundred seventy-four new pages?"

Nash responded, "Yes."

"How did you find so much additional information when you told me the last time we spoke that you had looked everywhere you could think of for any legally related documents, so it's not like there were any other places to look?"

Nash forced a grin. "Well, last time, I looked everywhere at the Chamber that would relate to Lovelace. For example, I looked through all our drives and our computer systems. I looked through all the desks of all our current employees. I looked through files related to our financial department, wherever I thought there might be some contracts connected to them. I looked through all our employees who worked in the membership division. In our storeroom I looked in every section I thought might have documents. In those areas where there should have been documents is where I looked."

Joel clarified, "Last time?"

Nash took a sip of water. "Correct."

Joel smiled. "So this time, where did you look?"

"This time, I looked through every single box in the storeroom."

Joel put his hand on the stack of new documents. "So you have now looked through every single place at the Chamber for documents that could relate to Lovelace and the Chamber."

"Yes."

Once again, Joel smiled. "And you have found for me every single document, correct?"

Nash looked extremely nervous and glanced at her council as she answered, "Correct."

This deposition was so important because the Chamber

had initially denied the existence of a Health Services Contract between Lovelace and the Chamber. After her first deposition, Andrea Nash found a signed 2004 Health Services Contract and a few related documents on top of a box in the storeroom. It was on top of documents from 2007. No other 2004 documents were in the box. The Chamber forwarded the newly found contract to Lovelace, who submitted it to the court. Up to this time, Lovelace had successfully remained hidden behind its wall of lawyers. But every word Andrea Nash spoke at her deposition ripped away a brick of the company's façade until Lovelace's misdeeds faced daylight.

The copy of the contract that was submitted to the court was a hodgepodge of several previously submitted documents and a copy of a signature page. The problem for Lovelace and the Chamber was that each page was date-stamped to eliminate the possibility of reproducing the same document or confusing similar documents. The copy supplied had date stamps from several previously submitted documents, which meant someone intentionally put the document together from several documents. Bill Webber wrote in the Plaintiff's Status Report to the Court in October 2009:

> Once the unthinkable premise was accepted, the rest became obvious. Never did we dream that Lovelace would actually submit a counterfeit contract to conceal the dispositive fact that there simply was no original signed contract. Never did we dream that Lovelace actually approved an earlier April 2004 Request for Treatment that was approved, and

then buried it because there is no way to unapprove a coverage approval. Never did we dream that the way Lovelace effected this "unapproval" was by returning the Maloneys' April insurance premium payment so as to "erase" coverage for that period.

Once we finally thought the unthinkable, what Lovelace secretly did to Zelphoe Maloney became almost deadly clear. Once that fraudulent die was cast, the fraud spread to a cover-up in the Maloneys' appeal to the superintendent of insurance. Once the superintendent upheld the denial of coverage under a nonexistent exclusion in a nonexistent contract, that fraud metastasized into the "fraud on the Court" . . . One of the first things counsel did was to request a copy of the group insurance policy—which they pointed out had not been reviewed in connection with the denial of coverage. By now, Lovelace was heavily invested in the misconduct that had already occurred. It had hidden the fact that there was no written contract and no written exclusion for experimental treatment from the Maloneys and the superintendent. Lovelace promised to furnish the contract to Maloney counsel. It simply didn't keep that promise—for over four years.

Instead, Lovelace filed a motion to dismiss the lawsuit—based upon an arbitration clause in the nonexistent contract/Handbook! When the Maloneys responded that the contract itself had not been produced, Lovelace withdrew the motion without comment. But, again it didn't produce the contract. Who would ever dream that the first motion in the lawsuit was based upon a contract that didn't exist? .. Every deposition taken until last month—after the counterfeit contract was discovered—has been tainted by the concealments and the continuing refusals of Lovelace to comply with this Court's discovery Order. In depositions taken in October and November 2009, we learned of four critical facts for the first time:

Although Lovelace Health Plan is a subdivision of a New Mexico corporation called Lovelace Health Systems, Inc., the Health Plan itself literally had no employees. Every person who worked for the insurance arm of the company was actually an employee of Ardent Health Systems, Inc., a foreign corporation not licensed in New Mexico.

The President of the Health Plan, Gayle Adams, knew virtually nothing about the lawsuit because it was turned over to "Compliance," which reports directly to Ardent's general counsel. Ms. Adams repeatedly testified that she would go to "Compliance" if one wanted to know crucial information about handling of the Maloney issues. No compliance documents have been produced.

While Lovelace has yet to produce contract files that concern Maloney, all of the original contract files of the Greater Albuquerque Chamber of Commerce concerning its Lovelace account have been destroyed during the pendency of this lawsuit.

Lovelace was paying the Chamber in the neighborhood of $180,000 per year as insurance "broker" commissions even though no significant brokerage services were being performed and even though no brokerage contract was signed until after the Maloneys hired counsel and filed this lawsuit. Sometimes these payments were made without there even being a licensed insurance agent.

The fraud in this case is not only upon the Maloneys . . . that was just the starting point and template for other victims of this fraud. When Lovelace concealed the April 2004 Request for Treatment and relied upon a nonexistent contract in the appeal to the superintendent of insurance, this became a case of fraud on the superintendent, who is charged with regulating insurance companies and protecting insured citizens. Had Lovelace "corrected the record" in front of the superintendent, his office would not have become embroiled in a five-year conflict that never should have happened. When Lovelace relied upon a nonexistent contract in framing its positions in this lawsuit, it subjected the Court itself to the fraud that began with the Maloneys. Lovelace built its defenses to the Maloneys' case on quicksand and now pretends that its house is not sinking and asks the Court to join it in that pretense. Over 20 depositions were taken by Plaintiffs in the blind, and over 20 motions were briefed on false foundations.

Now, however, it appears that the rights of over 400 businesses and over 1,000 other insured are implicated. It is no longer simply a question of whether Zelphoe Maloney was denied coverage under a nonexistent contractual "exclusion." It is no longer just about the missing Maloney documents. It's about all the Chamber-Lovelace contracts for all of the years—because all of those contracts seemed to have disappeared. Now, and since the last hearing, we discovered that the Greater Albuquerque Chamber of Commerce destroyed all of its original Lovelace contract files during the pendency of this lawsuit—and while the President of Lovelace was sitting on the Chamber's board of directors. Simultaneously, Lovelace itself has failed to produce records that could demonstrate whether Zelphoe Maloney got "special" treatment or whether this was the way Lovelace treated all of its 1,000 Chamber of Commerce insureds . . . One of the many problems here is that all of the Chamber's Lovelace contract files have vanished. (Luckily, copies of a few documents useful to Lovelace did show up in a dusty storage box that never had anything to do with contracts. The few documents that did show up from searching 100 storage boxes were all together and all right on top of 100 boxes). Under these circumstances, there is no evidence that this "evergreen" was ever planted in the first place.

Under the direction of Judge Sanchez, the truth about Lovelace and its practices was coming to light. Robert and I found it hard to believe the amount of deceit and corruption Lovelace was willing to engage in. But the more facts were revealed, the clearer the picture became. Bill, Bob, and Joel brought the blurred lines drawn by Lovelace into focus. It was a few weeks until the next hearing with Judge Sanchez, and our side was excited.

I was glad that we had not given up and surrendered in 2007, shortly after my kidney transplant. Lovelace had asked Bill to settle for $350,000, but by this time, Robert and I had nothing to lose. We no longer had Lovelace insurance, our finances were decimated, and we had signed a contract with our lawyers giving them 45 percent of any settlement plus expenses. Settling then would have done nothing for us and would have ended a majority of the investigation into Lovelace and the Office of Superintendent of Insurance. I could not in good conscience allow Lovelace and Serna to walk away and continue doing to other people what they had done to me.

Twenty-Four

Whose Side Are You on, God?

It was still dark the morning of December 7, 2009, when Robert and I got into our truck. A few flakes of snow fell.

"I hope the roads aren't too bad," Robert said as he started the truck. Before he could back out of the driveway, his phone rang. "Hey, Joel," Robert answered.

"Hey, Robert," Joel said, "don't worry about coming in. Court's been canceled due to snow."

"Snow? It's barely coming down here."

"I got here last night so I could set up for court early this morning. Bill has already turned back home. Have you left yet?"

"We were about ready to leave. Do you think it will open tomorrow?"

Robert could sense Joel's disappointment as he responded, "It doesn't work that way. We've lost this judge. There's no way he can hear this case before he retires. I think he was going to grant us some relief today. We will have to start over again, and I don't know if we'll get a decent judge."

I'm sure Nelson Franse breathed a big sigh of relief when he heard the news of the court closure. School was canceled as well, so we made the best of it with our children, building a snowman in the backyard that evening and making cookies and hot chocolate. It helped relieve the disappointment I felt over the delay.

The delay made me question is anything would go right for us in this case. At times like this, any normal person who looks up to the heavens and asks, "Why me?" I had a vague recollection of the Book of Job and looked up the verses later—the verses that I felt captured my feelings as Job addressed God about why he had been assaulted with so many tragedies, maladies, and setbacks:

> How many crimes and sins have I committed? Make me aware of my disobedience and my sin.
>
> Why do you hide your face from me nd consider me your enemy? Are you trying to make a fluttering leaf tremble or trying to chase dry husks?
>
> You write down bitter accusations against me. You make me suffer for the sins of my youth.
>
> You put my feet in shackles. You follow my trail by engraving marks on the soles of my feet. I am like worn-out wineskins, like moth-eaten clothes.
>
> (Job 13: 23-28)

Franse and Lovelace had stalled and delayed our case at every opportunity. Now, when it seemed we might catch a break, Mother Nature had joined in on Lovelace's side. The weather was not that bad. I had seen more severe storms that hadn't required Santa Fe to shut down. I now wonder if the closing of the court had more to do with Judge Sanchez retiring than Mother Nature. It would not surprise me to learn that the closure was ordered by someone high up in government trying to help Lovelace.

* * *

Judge Sanchez did not make any rulings on our case after that cancellation. He did, however, recommend that a new judge be appointed for our case.

Robert and I stood up as the bailiff announced Judge Sarah Singleton on June 23, 2010. I felt tense as she walked into the courtroom. She was in her early fifties, with salt-and-pepper hair and pale skin, and she carried herself in a no-nonsense way. I'm not sure if it was intuition or the comforting glance she sent our way as she sat down, but the tension I'd been feeling moments earlier disappeared.

Shortly after the proceedings began, a refreshing tone came from the judge's lips. "Okay, folks," she said, "I know you had a scheduling order before, so I'm not sure how much of this stuff we still need to go over, but the first thing that I put in my Rule 16 (B) scheduling order was a mandatory mediation settlement conference deadline. Have you scheduled the conference?"

Franse answered, "We have, Your Honor."

Once again, we had what appeared to be a favorable judge, and she was nowhere near ready to retire. Looking back, I feel that

Franse knew something of Judge Singleton. He didn't try any of his typical courtroom antics in her presence, just straightforward, "Yes, Your Honor," or "No, Your Honor." It was funny to see his character change. From this moment forward, Franse no longer attempted to stall depositions, or if he did, he disguised it well. Instead, he focused on preparing for trial.

The only deceitful thing I noticed he did was to send every piece of information he had on my case to our attorneys when Judge Singleton requested he do so. The problem was that he sent every scrap, whether it was pertinent or not. Joel later told me this was a tactic used to overwhelm opposing counsel and confuse an issue with too much information.

But it was a huge blunder on Franse's part. Joel meticulously took apart every document and used the information to piece together the scenario behind my denial of coverage and the cover-up that had ensued. The details of the cover-up were so profound that even Franse would have had difficulty defending the actions of Lovelace. When the time came for depositions, Joel and Bill demolished the witnesses that Lovelace provided. Some of the witnesses I felt sorry for, but others showed their true natures when cornered under oath.

Another issue that Joel discussed with Robert and me was what to present to the jury. It seemed Judge Singleton was going to give us our trial, but our case was complex, and Lovelace's antics sometimes seemed unbelievable. Joel was afraid the jury might get lost in the evidence. The most interesting portion of the case Joel decided to leave out was what he believed drove the financial reason for the denial in the first place back in 2004. He was convinced it was a major reason why Lovelace needed to keep all expensive treatments, like my $100,000 transplant, performed and billed in-house.

Joel explained how Lovelace operated and how billing and collection practices were managed. Ardent Health Services, which now owned Lovelace, was set to go public months before this lawsuit was filed. Profitability was the key between a great initial public offering and a poor initial public offering.

Our attorneys had discovered Ardent's practice of "double revenue" during discovery. All Lovelace's billings were counted as income on the supply side of the business, while all the collections were counted as income on the collection side of the business, even though most of the billings were in-house. That is, Lovelace logged collection from itself. The company would count revenue twice for the same service—once when it billed for the service and then again when it paid itself. This practice made Lovelace appear substantially more profitable than it was. Consider the effect on an initial public offering.

Through Ardent's spokesperson, Shea Davis, Lovelace tried to explain away their actions:

> Lovelace Sandia Health Systems Inc. overstated its pre-tax earnings by $20 million in 2003 and 2004 and is moving to correct the misstatements, the Albuquerque company's parent said late Tuesday.
>
> The overstatements were the result of improper accounting entries that were discovered earlier this year by the system's parent, the Nashville, Tenn.-based Ardent Health Services . . .

The misstatements did not involve fraud and did not involve a third party, Ardent said in a news release on the matter. The misstatements involved the 191,000-member Lovelace Health Plan and its system of hospitals and clinics.

The health plan's expenses were often underreported, while revenues for the system's six hospitals were often overstated, Davis said.

(*New Mexico Business Weekly*, December 1, 2004)

Joel concurred with my deduction: If Lovelace had done my transplant in-house, they could show $100,000 on the coverage side of the plan when they billed the provider side of Lovelace and show another $100,000 on the provider side when they paid the other side of Lovelace. That would show a net of $200,000. If Lovelace let me go out of network—to the University of Massachusetts or Northwestern—the books would show a $100,000 expense. That would not look good for a company trying to look profitable for a public offering. With this in mind, it's not surprising that Ardent occasionally postponed submitting its financial records to the Securities and Exchange Commission.

Twenty-Five

Fire and Ice

Judge Singleton had ordered us into mediation with Lovelace. Joel wanted to keep on track for a jury trial and accepted Lovelace's offer to host the mediation but informed Franse that we would continue with the scheduled depositions as planned. Joel expected the upcoming depositions to reveal further proof of Lovelace's deception and fraud, and he had little faith that Lovelace would negotiate in good faith.

Dr. Harold Sunderman, one of Lovelace's medical directors, was in charge of the approval process for cases that reached his desk. From what I witnessed, Sunderman was the gatekeeper for out-of-network funding for medically necessary procedures. We believe that Lovelace tried to keep all procedures in-house and avoid out-of-network payments at all costs. Just before Sunderman's deposition, tension pulsed in the room. Seated across from Robert and me was the man who had ordered the reversal of the approval for the stem cell transplant. My husband is a gentleman, but I could tell he would have loved to give Sunderman a solid whack on the jaw. Robert's evident rage did not affect Sunderman as he calmly poured himself a glass of water and leaned back in his seat, cool and confident.

Joel proceeded to ask Sunderman, "Doc, isn't it true that the plan has, both by its contract and by regulation, five days from the day it receives a request to approve or deny the claim?"

Sunderman responded, "I believe that is correct."

"So on April 27, 2004, the first request was made?"

"Yes."

"Let's just look at this. We should see a denial of this first request sometime in five days, shouldn't we?"

Sunderman looked puzzled. "I would assume so."

Joel smiled. "And Doctor, if we don't have a denial of the claim, then by regulation, isn't it approved?" Joel had hit hard at Lovelace's premise that it followed all regulations in my denial process. "Okay," he continued. "This is dated April 27, 2004. Right?"

"Uh-huh."

"All right. Doctor, we've got another one that is dated May 7, 2004. Right?"

"Yes."

The tension was building. "Okay. One thing I want to make sure is clear, though, Doc: whatever happened, we're either missing documents, or Lovelace dropped the ball on approving or denying this claim in a timely manner. Right?"

Sunderman questioned, "Are you referring to your compilation of exhibits that you put together today, or are you referring to the official appeals file in this case?"

"I'd refer to anything. If you have another document that shows that there was something denied within five days of April 27, 2004, or five days from May 7, 2004, I'd like to see it."

"Well, certainly, one possibility is missing documents. Certainly, one possibility is that the timeline was not met. And I suspect there are probably other possibilities too, but I can't think of them right now."

"Doc, I'd like to look at 58, but I'm going to start with 59 because that's where your signature is. Isn't that your signature dated May 17, 2004?"

"Yes."

"And that's a denial?"

"Yes."

Joel continued, "Does it appear that a fax has either come or gone to Intracorp at ten fifty-four on the seventeenth and at the top also May 17, 2004, at eight forty-seven? Do you see that?"

"Yes."

Sometime thereafter, during the deposition, Joel asked, "Can we take a short break?"

"We are off the record."

I stared at the man who had ordered my death sentence. Sunderman stared back at me, silent. Although he did not respond with words, his face said, *She's determined not to let this go.* Joel politely asked me to sit down and wait for the deposition to resume. Then he turned his focus on Sunderman.

The deposition really hurt me. As I sat and listened, I wondered how a doctor could intentionally deny someone's life. Then I looked into his eyes. He was afraid. That brought me some hope that he had some semblance of emotion. Joel articulated this beautifully in a letter he drafted for the mediator, William Madison, on December 7, 2010:

> Mrs. Maloney's Lovelace-employed doctor ordered a bone marrow transplant ("BMT") on April 27, 2004, and sent it to Lovelace's health services division for authorization or denial. Lovelace forwarded it to a subcontractor who exclusively handled Lovelace transplants, and that vendor failed to issue a notice of denial within the five-day deadline required under the statute. Mrs. Maloney did not receive a denial of any BMT until May 17, 2004 . . . Dr. Sunderman, the Lovelace chief medical director, received a recommendation from a subcontractor at about 10:45 a.m. on Monday, May 17. Sunderman signed a form denying the BMT within seven minutes of receiving it. He signed the denial form, which the subcontractor had prepared, and didn't bother to give even one basis for the denial. He checked a pre-printed box that said, "deny." That's it. He didn't even check one of the thirteen pre-printed boxes explaining his reasoning, much less write an explanation . . .
>
> Here's what preceded that seven-minute death sentence. The front-line nurse of the transplant subcontractor called a medical director for the subcontractor and explained the request. Less than an hour later, that nurse wrote down the names of three journal articles, which he said supported denial (though one

was only written in Japanese) . . . That same day, the nurse for the subcontractor called Dr. Sunderman at 5:55 p.m. They spoke on the phone, and Sunderman "agreed" with the denial decision. Thus, Sunderman made this life-and-death decision in about five minutes on a Friday afternoon having never seen a single article, never talked to another doctor, never consulted a specialist, never consulted his "new technology" committee. He then re-confirmed that decision in seven minutes on a Monday morning.

Dr. Sunderman's deposition was still fresh in my mind on October 13, 2009, when I entered the Rodey Law Firm to conduct a continuation of my 2005 deposition. It was my turn to explain why Lovelace should not have denied me the bone marrow transplant. Bill Webber met me downstairs and escorted me up to the conference room. Robert was going to be a little late. I was nervous, not because of the deposition but because of how I feared Nelson Franse would treat me based on past experiences with him.

This time, we were meeting in a dedicated conference room instead of a repurposed storage closet. It was stocked with refreshments. As I sat and listened to Bill review a couple of items he thought would be mentioned, Brian Brack walked in. He was well dressed, minus his coat. "I'm covering for Nelson," he said. "He had another matter to attend to."

When I heard that, a great burden was lifted. The deposition started as usual, with basic questions to address the obvious: "Can you state your name, please?" Soon after the formalities, Robert quietly walked in and sat next to me.

Brack continued, "Did you understand if there were any limits on the insurance that you first received back in 1991?"

I answered, "No. I didn't know there should be any kind of limit on health insurance according to somebody's life or health. There shouldn't be."

"So you believe that it should cover everything related to your health?"

"Yes."

"Without limitations?"

"Yes."

"What is the basis of that belief, ma'am? Why do you have that?"

"Because we are talking about human lives. I'm a human being. I'm not a car."

Brack was polite, but his words meant business. He was not going to hold back. "Do you understand that the Lovelace Health Plan takes the position that experimental treatments are not covered?"

"No. At the time, I didn't know that because they covered IVIG."

"At some point, did you understand that was their position?"

"After I appealed, I heard the 'experimental' word over and over and over, but if they approved one, I didn't understand why they wouldn't approve the other one. I think it was the difference in the amount of money the treatments cost. To me, it was more about money than anything else, more than saving people or giving me treatment. If they were to give it to me, they would have to give it to somebody else."

"Let me make sure I understand what you're saying. You

believe that the health plan approved the IVIG treatment and not the bone marrow transplant because the bone marrow transplant was more expensive?"

I was a bit confused by the direction of the questions, but I held to my belief. "Yes."

"Is it your understanding, ma'am, that you were not referred to or seen by a heart specialist—"

"No."

"—because of the expense?"

"I think—it seems to me Dr. O'Sullivan was saving money for the insurance, or he was scared, or he was getting a bonus. I'm not exactly sure at the time what it was, but I knew something was wrong."

"What do you think he was scared of?"

"Lovelace, maybe."

"In what way?"

"Losing his job."

"For what?"

"Giving me the treatment that I needed."

"Is it your belief that he did not refer you to a heart specialist because he was worried about the expense or his job?"

"It seems that way. When I went to Northwestern, Dr. Oyama was furious. He asked why they hadn't taken care of all these problems . . . All this should have been addressed a long, long time ago. That is the reason I am saying this about Lovelace and O'Sullivan, because by the time I went to Northwestern, my heart was twice its normal size, with fluid around the lungs and the heart. There is no way O'Sullivan would have not known that. There was no way. I felt it myself. There is no way."

It appeared that Brack was pleased with my responses, and that concerned me. After a short break, he continued, saying, "You mentioned the word 'heartless.' Do you think the Lovelace Health Plan is heartless?"

"What do you think?"

"I am asking what you think, ma'am."

"What everybody else would think. I know you would think the same thing that I do. You don't have to ask me that. You already know."

"Do you believe that a bone marrow transplant for the treatment of lupus in June of 2004 was not experimental?"

"No."

"It is your understanding that it was not experimental or that it was?"

"I'm proof that it is not experimental. I'm alive. Can you see me? Do you think that was experimental? I'm alive."

The deposition was difficult, but at the end of the day, I think even Brack was beginning to doubt his defense of Lovelace. I'm glad I wasn't on the other side of the table questioning a survivor like Brack had to. Only the most cold-hearted person could have come away from our encountered unscathed.

Twenty-Six

The Price Tag on My Life

It had been three years since I'd seen Dr. Frank O'Sullivan. As Robert and I waited for him to enter the deposition room on September 1, 2009, Joel was reviewing documents on the table. When he walked in, I saw a man who looked years younger than the last time I had seen him. His hair was not quite as white, and his wrinkled face was smoother. It looked as though he'd had a face-lift.

After we took our seats, O'Sullivan was sworn in. Joel wasted no time, asking questions about his compensation package with Lovelace and how it changed once Ardent took over operations. At this point, I was not sure what Joel was getting at. His questions seemed off-topic as if he were grasping at straws. Then he changed direction. He glanced out the window, grinned, and asked O'Sullivan to look at Exhibit 4.

"The purpose of writing this letter," he said, "was to tell

the licensing board that you had not been sued for malpractice, and the plaintiff had not alleged that you did anything wrong. Is that correct?"

"Well, more or less. The idea was to be sure the board was fully informed of any actions that I'd been involved in at all."

Joel clarified, "Well, the intent was to fully inform the board, correct?"

"I think my intent was simply to give the board a heads-up."

"Okay. Doctor, I guess the thing that I'm a little bit surprised about is that in paragraph 137 of the amended complaint, where there's an allegation that Dr. O'Sullivan took over Mrs. Maloney's primary care and failed to have her evaluated by other specialists or to consult properly with the same, besides it you've written, 'Bullshit, this is slanderous.' Correct?"

"Correct."

"And then you've written on the other side of that, 'I resent this. Who is better qualified than an experienced board-certified rheumatologist?' Correct?"

"Correct."

"Do you believe that the things you have written on page 26 of the amended complaint, Exhibit 4, are consistent with the explanation you gave in the letter to the licensing board on June 21, 2006?"

O'Sullivan squirmed in his seat and looked away from us.

"You may answer, Doctor."

"What if I don't want to?"

"Sorry, Doctor, it's just—you have to answer."

Joel had gotten under his skin. Then Joel switched to the

support O'Sullivan had with regard to my stem cell transplant. Joel asked him to read from his notes.

"Well, what I wrote here was that I spoke to Robert, told him I took Dr. Traynor's call yesterday and told her I don't think the patient's lupus is now affecting any organs except kidneys and occasionally joints. Dr. Traynor has rejected Zelphoe as a stem cell transplant candidate. It was not my decision."

Joel asked, "You just provided the facts?"

"I told Dr. Traynor that I didn't think that she had other organ involvement."

"Doctor, do you think that prudence would have dictated that you check her heart, check her lungs to see whether there was any other organ involvement?"

"I really can't respond to that question in terms of prudence."

"Did you ever consider sending Mrs. Maloney to a nephrologist?"

"I'm sure I considered it, but I never thought it was necessary."

"Doctor, are you aware that in March of 2005, less than sixty days after you last saw Mrs. Maloney, she went to Northwestern and showed up there with cardiomegaly (enlarged heart) and pleural effusion (excess fluid around the lungs) and some cardiac effusion (fluid around the heart)?"

"No."

"Were you aware that in July of 2005, five months after she last saw you, she had an EKG that showed that she had an infarct of undetermined age?"

"No."

"Did she have any cardiovascular risk factors, Doctor?"

"Well . . ."

"Okay. Mrs. Maloney showed up in September of 2004, Doctor, in Dr. Gieri's office, saying that she felt like she had a balloon exerting pressure around her heart. Did you ever see that note?"

"Not that I recall."

"His analysis is chest pain of uncertain etiology. Do you see that?"

"I see it."

"Is that something that should have been sent to a cardiologist?"

At this point, we can take a step back and see what other physicians really thought of Dr. Frank O'Sullivan's handling of my case. In a deposition conducted on October 10, 2009, expert witness Timothy Hammond, MD, summed up Dr. O'Sullivan's practices.

Franse asked, "So when is a rheumatologist who is comfortable treating a patient who has lupus—because they're trained to treat such patients, correct?"

Hammond responded, "Yes, sir."

"Okay. And they're also trained to treat patients with lupus nephritis, too, correct?"

"In part. The lupus nephritis I see is almost always referred to a nephrologist."

"Okay. So a rheumatologist has this training to treat patients with lupus, correct?"

"Correct."

"And they have training to treat at least some patients with lupus nephritis, correct?"

"Correct."

"And they need to use the training that they've received as rheumatologists to know whenever they're outside their comfort zone, they need to refer a patient with lupus nephritis to a nephrologist, correct?"

"Not correct because you've made one assumption—"

Franse looks puzzled. "Okay."

"—And that is, I think a rheumatologist looking at a rising creatinine and blood pressure elevated on many occasions and increasing proteinuria (excess proteins in the urine) should be seeing warning signs that they either need to intervene more aggressively with renal management or ask for help. I don't see adequate documentation on the chart that Dr. O'Sullivan understands that this renal situation is going to the devil in a hand basket, and that's what bothers me."

"Okay."

"If he had given appropriate care, and the patient got all the care they needed, I'd have no problem with him managing it. What bothers me is that's not what I'm seeing here. That's why I have a problem with it."

"Okay."

"If he had done a thousand lupus nephritis cases and managed their Cytoxan, and he did fine, no problem. My problem is when he's saying he's in his comfort zone and the patients are not getting what they need. That's when I have a problem."

"Okay. So it's not that he needed to refer, it's that she didn't get appropriate treatment, is that right?"

"Right. And like I told you, there are two ways in medicine always: you can do it yourself, if you know how to do it and you're watching the outcome, or you can ask for help. What bothers me here is he didn't ask for help, self-evident progression, and we're not intervening appropriately."

"Okay."

"So I actually have a problem with a rheumatologist managing lupus nephritis. I have a problem when I see the disease getting out of hand and appropriate things not happening."

In depositions, Joel discovered that O'Sullivan was the only doctor to receive a bonus for the period, including several years prior to when I filed my case in 2004 and up until the mediation in 2010. Joel referenced this in the letter he wrote to the mediator, William Madison. In several depositions, Joel tried to get an explanation for the bonus, but no one, including O'Sullivan, could or would explain it. Frank O'Sullivan had accepted a $30,000 bonus check shortly after he suggested to Dr. Ann Traynor that I was not an acceptable candidate for transplant. I still cannot fathom this level of betrayal. Robert was right: Lovelace had placed a value on my life.

After his testimony, it seemed that Lovelace officials turned on O'Sullivan. In a conversation I overheard between Nelson Franse and my lawyers, Franse blatantly suggested that this case should be a malpractice suit against my former rheumatologist, not against Lovelace.

A friend of mine who worked in the business office at Lovelace confirmed news reports about Ardent's takeover of Lovelace. They fired or accepted resignations from a large number of doctors. This furthered my belief that Lovelace viewed doctors as cash machines instead of health partners. According to her this was caused by the new pay plan Ardent was implementing, where doctors could earn bonuses for seeing more patients for shorter times and not referring procedures out of the Lovelace network. The one good thing that came out of my experience with O'Sullivan was the privilege of being treated by Drs. Oyama and Burt, and the wonderful Kim Young.

My dilemma with O'Sullivan reminded me of an old Western where a price is placed on some innocent cowboy's head just because he's "in the way." If the reward is high enough, people with no scruples will come out of the woodwork to kill him.

Twenty-Seven

The Case of the Dubious Expert Witness

In a court case, is it possible to over-think a scenario? To be so overconfident of the outcome of a discussion that you let your guard down? We had experienced this early in our case in regard to Bob Mayfield predicting Judge Garcia's actions in handling the deposition of Eric Serna. But who could predict the testimony of a witness that effectively sabotages your case?

Nelson Franse discovered, to his dismay, that a sharp mind and impeccable people skills do not compensate for common sense. This is what I recall about Joel's description of the deposition of Dr. Brian Heller, whom Lovelace had tapped as an expert witness.

"Okay, Doctor, let's say you were in charge of a patient . . . such as Mrs. Maloney . . . with signs of renal failure . . . and you have read her file, correct?" Joel asked.

Dr. Heller replied, "Yes, I have."

Joel continued, "With a patient with renal problems like Mrs. Maloney, would you recommend IVIG?"

Franse stood up. "Objection. Hypothetical!"

Heller answered, "No."

"And why is that?"

"Because it is well documented that IVIG causes kidney damage."

Joel responded, "In your opinion, should Dr. O'Sullivan and the Lovelace medical director have known about these risks to Mrs. Maloney's kidneys?"

"Yes. They should have been well aware."

"So, according to everything we've discussed today, you are saying there was no breach of contract, bad faith, or malpractice?"

Heller paused for a beat, thinking. "Well, now that you put it that way ... there was bad faith, medical malpractice, and a breach of contract ..."

Franse perked up, and Joel and Bill looked at each other in disbelief. Franse slapped his hand on the table. "Stop! Can we go off the record? This deposition's over!"

Joel fired back, "What do you mean it's over? He's your malpractice expert."

"I know damn well whose expert he is, but I'm recusing him right now!" Franse responded before turning to walk away.

Joel lowered his voice. "You have the right to recuse him, but I'm just going to call him an expert for the plaintiffs. Your client's lust for profit affected everyone in a bad way."

It must have become resoundingly evident to Franse that his defense was unraveling. His own paid witnesses could see right through Lovelace's practices. I did not think Franse was inherently evil like some of those involved in the case seemed to be. Until my attorneys exposed Lovelace's true nature, I think Franse believed he was doing his job by protecting Lovelace from frivolous litigation. I never had a chance to discuss with Franse his thoughts during this ordeal, but the internal struggle between humanity and work objectives must have become excruciating.

Joel would not relent.

Sometimes, you don't realize the danger you are in until someone else points it out. And even when you stare at the evidence, you can't believe what has happened, or why information was withheld. Some say ignorance is bliss. I say ignorance is deadly.

I was reluctant to travel in late summer of 2010 for an evaluation of my current heart health. Still, Joel said this doctor in Hollywood, California, was the top cardiologist in the region. Dr. Shapiro was going to be deposed as an expert witness, and he said he would be more comfortable if he actually saw me as a patient instead of relying solely on the reports from Lovelace.

When Shapiro walked in, Robert and I were pleasantly surprised by his optimistic attitude. "Mrs. Maloney, it is a pleasure to finally meet you and your husband in person. I know quite a bit about your medical history from studying your records, but a good old-fashioned exam is the best approach. Besides, your being here in and of itself is a miracle."

At the time our conversation began, I thought he meant the fact that I had received successful stem cell and kidney transplants, but my medical chart told a sinister tale. Under Lovelace's care, I had not only experienced an enlarged heart, but Shapiro also revealed evidence of a heart attack I experienced in 2005, a heart attack that Lovelace had not disclosed. Evidence of Lovelace's willingness to provide substandard care and conceal it was mounting.

For several years, I was under the care of a single rheumatologist, Frank O'Sullivan. Shapiro reinforced the opinions of Drs. Burt and Oyama at Northwestern said that I should have been provided with a cardiologist, a nephrologist, a pulmonologist, a rheumatologist, and an endocrinologist. It seemed that Lovelace or someone working at Lovelace allowed only a rheumatologist to manage all of my medical conditions. Only on a few occasions did O'Sullivan refer me to another specialist. This action no doubt kept costs down and made it easier to control treatment recommendations. It was now crystal clear to me that the bottom line had taken precedence over human life.

Twenty-Eight

Unwavering Resolve

Some lawyers build a career on confusing issues, clouding details, and raising questions about a person's integrity. There are those few people of character for whom attacks simply fall by the wayside, leaving only the sting of truth. It is people like Dr. Richard Burt who ensure that the vulnerable have a voice.

Robert relayed to me his discussion with Joel about the deposition of Dr. Richard Burt on December 10, 2010. Dr. Oyama was in Tokyo, so Dr. Burt had agreed to the deposition in his absence, since he had overseen my entire transplant evaluation and procedure. According to Joel, Franse made every attempt to distort Dr. Burt's testimony. But when Franse asked if he could describe the details behind my stem cell transplant, Franse got an earful.

Richard Burt perked up. "You bet I can. When Mrs. Maloney arrived, it took a group of specialists a month to get her strong enough for the transplant. She was bordering on the need for dialysis; she had fibrosis in both lungs, and there was scarring in the heart. It was a miracle she made it at all. And to top it off, she only had a single doctor, a rheumatologist, managing all her conditions. She should have had three specialists at minimum. Need I continue, Mr. Franse?"

Franse stepped back to his seat and flipped through some papers on the table, then faced Dr. Burt. "No, that's enough. I know that previous to the last question, you said you didn't experiment on Mrs. Maloney, but is that not the nature of a phase-two clinical trial, to experiment as to the validity of a proposed treatment?"

Burt looked straight at Franse, opened his hand, and poked it with his index finger as he exclaimed, "You know Lovelace's definition of experimental: M,O,N,E,Y. Money! Mrs. Maloney is the victim here. I don't care how many times you ask me or how many times you spin the question, and my answer will always be that I never experimented on Mrs. Maloney or any other patient. We have been developing sound protocols for this procedure for over twenty years, and I, as well as others, have published findings in several accredited publications. There, do you understand now?"

Joel conducted most of the remainder of the deposition; Franse had become gun-shy about asking further questions. As an expert witness, Richard Burt was entitled to compensation for his testimony. At the end of the deposition, he took Joel aside and asked that the payment, which amounted to thousands of dollars, be given to me. He also asked that Joel make sure Lovelace did not delay the transaction, because he knew we were in desperate need and he did not need the money. I was so grateful to Dr. Burt for his compassion, both at the hospital and also when I was no longer his patient. When I worked through the emotion, I thought, *The kids will have Christmas after all.*

The humbling news of the gift from Dr. Richard Burt came on December 13, 2010. But it was overshadowed by a call I received from my mother. My baby brother had been murdered at the young age of thirty-seven. He'd been walking down the street with a couple of friends when a figure stepped out from behind an SUV and demanded, "Give me your money." One of his friends turned and ran. The person shot him down. My brother and the other friend immediately turned to run, but before they could get into full stride, shots rang out, and they both bled to death before an ambulance could arrive. Combined, the three had less than fifty dollars on them. There are many things I do not understand, but I do know in my heart and my head the precious value of life.

Twenty-Nine

Stress

Stress changes a person. However the combination of physical with mental stress can alter both health and the health of relationships. The Lovelace litigation amped up tensions and anxiety for all involved. We were stressed to the point of possibly causing our allies to turn on one another. This is how I remember one of the last meetings Robert and I had with our attorneys.

I sat and listened as everyone discussed the case. They acted as if I were not in the room and had no say in the matter. After hours of listening to lawyers and interested parties, I made a gut-wrenching decision that threatened to implode the entire process.

Bill commented, "I think it's decent to try and avoid court."

Robert added, "But do you think they're serious? Last time, they came back later and said they didn't have an approval."

"I understand, but we need to find a solution," Bill added.

Robert continued, "I'm not sure if we can give up just yet."

Everyone fell silent as I stood up. *Is that all you care about?* I thought. *I lost my kidneys and my youth, and now these bastards are going to walk away like nothing happened. I can't take this anymore. You accepted this case. And now you are just complaining. No more.*

"You know what? I'm sick of this!" I was exploding emotionally. "I don't know how many times you've mentioned how much money you've spent on this lawsuit. I don't want to be around rude people!" I looked right at Bill's wife and asked, "Do you know how it makes me feel every time you mention how much you've spent on this? I'm tired of listening to you complain about wasted time and money. I've lost everything, everything but the price on my head. Is that all you care about?"

Robert comforted me as the rest of the people in the room exchanged pained glances. They were at a loss for words. "All of you, just keep any money!" I said. "I'm leaving, and I hope I never see you rude people again!" At that moment, I just wanted to leave and never come back; every word seemed like mumbling. Then, my mind went blank.

Joel stood up. "Robert, what's going on?"

Robert took my hand and said, "I'm with Gabby. This was never about the money." Then, he escorted me to the elevators.

In reality, I wanted to go to court. And before my outburst, I believe Joel did, too. I could tell by his puzzled expression that he was tired of the drawn-out litigation but was not quite ready to let go. He had worked on this case for years and was as prepared for court as I have seen anyone be prepared for anything in my life. It just seemed court would have to be the final solution. The last step Joel would have to take before trial would be practicing in front of a mock jury. Robert's decision and mine could change the dynamic of our coalition's relationship forever.

When the elevator door opened in the parking garage, all my bottled-up emotions released an unstoppable flow of tears. Relief had finally come. Robert wrapped his arms around me and told me not to worry. Eventually, the same thoughts that kept running through my mind came out in words. "The criminals are getting away with it. Richardson and Serna are getting away with it. They're all getting away with it! Judge Garcia got a promotion to the Court of Appeals, and Lujan was a congressman. Almost everyone who tried to help me was ruined—Castellano, Chavez, Baca, and for what?"

Robert gave me a tired smile. "Hon, we gave them the fight of their lives. The news coverage about our situation sparked the FBI investigation that probably led to Richardson's withdrawal from consideration for Obama's commerce secretary. Serna was removed as superintendent of insurance. Joe Ruiz is in prison, and Ardent couldn't take Lovelace public. I'm sorry, hon, but I'm tired."

I looked into Robert's crying eyes. "It's okay. I understand."

Robert kissed me gently, helped me into the truck, and then walked around to get in. Before he could close his door, the second elevator door opened, and Joel stepped out. Joel approached the truck with a look of concern.

"I'm sorry you feel that way," he said, "but it's been over six years, and there could be another three years of appeals even if we do win the case. Robert, what do I tell them?"

Robert turned to me, and we locked eyes for a moment. I

lowered my head in silence, and Robert turned back to Joel. "Do what you feel is right. We'll support your decision."

Robert closed the door, then reached up and gently took my face and turned it toward him. Before he could speak, I asked, "Why?"

Robert shook his head. "I don't care anymore."

I was hurt that only Joel had come to apologize and see how I was. It would have meant a great deal if Bill and his wife had checked on me as well, but maybe they were unable to do so for whatever reason. Stress is powerful. And its power effectively broke the unity of our coalition.

The main thing I learned from dealing with extreme stress is that sometimes, we need to step back and analyze the situation. Individuals can lose focus on what really matters. People can be easily distracted by stress. But stress can be overcome by determination—and by taking a look around at the genuine care that other people have for us.

Thirty

Forgiveness

After dozens of depositions, additional specialists' reviews of my medical history, and weeks short of Judge Singleton's deadline mandate for mediation to take place, Lovelace invited us for negotiation.

It was a cold January day in 2011. The mediation was to start at one o'clock in the afternoon. Bill and his wife, Joel, Robert, and I met in the hotel restaurant of the Hyatt Hotel at 11:30 for lunch. After we ordered, Franse and a team of lawyers and insurance executives walked in and took a table across the room from us. I wasn't sure of Franse's motive as he walked over to our table. Bill and Joel stood up and shook hands with him as he greeted us. "Are we ready for the mediation?" he asked.

Robert stood, and Franse reached to shake his hand. Robert accepted Franse's hand, squeezed it hard, and pulled him until the lawyer's face was an inch from his. Franse leaned back as

Robert said loudly, "I'm sick of this bullshit. You will treat us with respect." He let go of Franse's hand, and the Lovelace attorney took a step back. The rest of the table watched in anticipation while our attorneys struggled to hold back smiles.

In a sincere tone, Franse responded, "Mr. Maloney, I apologize. I had no idea you felt that way." Without skipping a beat, Robert took a step toward Franse and said, "You mean like when my wife was crying in pain while giving her deposition, and you sat across the table with your boots on the desk, reading a magazine?"

Franse shook his head, seemingly searching for a response, looking at everyone at our table and people from other tables who had begun to whisper among themselves.

After an awkward moment, Franse excused himself. "Like I said, Mr. Maloney, I'm sorry. I'll see everyone upstairs." Then Franse walked away.

Before our attorneys escorted us to the mediation, Bill wanted to take a quick puff. Joel remarked to Bill's wife, "Smoking might be affecting Bill."

I commented, "Lung cancer—"

No sooner had those words come out than Bill's wife shot back without looking at me, "It's nobody's business."

I was surprised that the wife of an attorney who fought for proper health care would respond in such a way. I had nearly died twice, through no fault of my own, and it hurt me to see someone possibly have to deal with something as serious as lung cancer. Robert and I awkwardly remained quiet and waited for Bill to come back inside.

Six years of failed litigation, years of hospitalization, the loss of our business, and moving our family from the house that had been our home for a decade—it all ended in a conference room in the Rodey Law Firm's two-floor suite atop the Bank of Albuquerque Building.

Closure is something that must be weighed against justice. My life had been dragged through a desert of cactus. The scales had shifted many times as the number of lies Lovelace tried to cover up was revealed. At one point, I would have settled for the stem cell transplant alone, and at other times, I wanted everybody involved at Lovelace, the Chamber of Commerce, and the New Mexico state government thrown in jail for what they had put me through. In the end, the torture of mediation had shifted the scales for Robert and me in favor of closure.

I cried the entire three-hour drive back home after the mediation. At one point, about ten o'clock at night, I looked out the passenger-side window into the dark sky. A feeling of peace filled me as I remembered the good things about my baby brother. At that moment, a barrage of falling stars shot through the sky. I like to think it was a final farewell from my brother, who loved me so much—his way of telling me he was watching out for me and that everything was going to be all right. In our last conversation, he said, "Keep going. You're strong."

I am alive. People from all walks of life joined in my rescue. My family is intact. I don't need to worry about Serna, judges, lawsuits, or Lovelace. My gratitude runs deep—for the nurses who checked my blood pressure, my attorneys, the astronaut who funded my stem cell transplant, and the man and his family who donated his kidney to me after his death—but I feel the fight is far from over. People like me are vulnerable, and that haunts me.

My life came at a cost—a sellout, if you will. Others may not see it as such, only that I was a woman who needed resolution to a dilemma years in the making. That is true. But a deal with the devil—Lovelace—is also a curse. It is a curse of knowing that other people might have to suffer a similar ordeal yet may not have the good fortune I experienced. Their result would be burying their loved ones prematurely. My concern for them will live on as long as I breathe, and I solemnly vow to expose anyone I can who uses greed to profit at the expense of the helpless.

In the end, I forgave everyone who willingly hurt me, as well as those who were used by others to unknowingly hurt me. At times I indeed wanted to sulk in pity or anger, but the realization that I can hold my children, kiss my husband, and witness the birth of our first grandchild has forged my desire not to waste another minute of life. I have gained a new faith that the legal system can work and that a cold-hearted cynic like Nelson Franse can develop a conscience.

But most important of all, I witnessed the love and concern of everyday people—people who willingly put themselves and their careers in jeopardy to help a dying woman. Ultimately, it has become clear to me that greed, especially the desire of corporate officers to produce exorbitant profits, affects everything around us. Yet the compassion and actions of even one person can tilt the scales from death to life.

Epilogue

Bob Mayfield died a short time after we settled our case. He was the youngest eighty-something person I ever met and a true warrior for justice all the way to the end. I believe Bob was hanging on for this case to settle, like a father looking after his child. Bill Webber has also committed his life to helping people in similar situations as mine. He is writing a book that outlines several cases he became familiar with during his extensive legal career. Joel Newton still practices law in New Mexico but feels shunned by other attorneys who exploited the corrupt system that was exposed due to our lawsuit. It was disclosed to me that, in some cases, the superintendent of insurance had the authority to negotiate settlements involving insurance companies. Lawyers on good terms with Eric Serna got the best deals. I hope that lawyers no longer have an inside person like Eric Serna with which to negotiate lucrative settlements.

I have had limited contact with Linda Peeno and wish her the very best. Joe Castellano, a dear friend, died October 12, 2018.

E. Shirley Baca works in community services in Las Cruces, New Mexico. Kim Young still works at Northwestern in Chicago. Dr. Richard Burt is currently practicing medicine at Northwestern. Dr. Yu Oyama is practicing medicine at Northwestern. I have lost touch with Dr. Ann Traynor. Mike Gallagher has retired from The Albuquerque Journal. Judge Sanchez is retired from the First Judicial District Court and still practices law in Santa Fe, New Mexico. Judge Singleton retired from the First Judicial District Court and passed away July 4th, 2019.

As I bring this story to a close, I believe the people involved have moved on. The New Mexico Public Regulation Commission has changed from a five-commissioned elected board to a three-commissioner board appointed by the Governor. The Superintendent of Insurance is now a separate entity from the PRC. Nelson Franse still practices law in Albuquerque. After talking with Joel, I feel that Franse views plaintiffs in a whole new way than he did before he took the case with Lovelace. I am hopeful he views them as people, not just the opposition. Dr. Frank O'Sullivan teaches medicine in New Mexico. Dr. Harold Sunderman is now a Cardiologist in Ruidoso, New Mexico. Judge Timothy Garcia retired from the New Mexico Court of Appeals in 2018. Joe Ruiz has been released from prison. Bill Richardson was implicated in the Jeffery Epstein incident by Giuffre. Richardson died in his sleep on September 1, 2023. Ben Ray Lujan is a US Senator from New Mexico. Eric Serna took full retirement from New Mexico and is a lobbyist for the insurance industry.

After the ordeal, I found myself in an awkward state of mind. Our family traveled to Las Vegas in March 2011 for a well-deserved family break. The twins were arguing in the back seat, Veronica kept staring out the window with no expression, Otis and Bridgette had earbuds in, listening to music, and my salt-and-pepper-haired husband drove on. Where had my youth gone? I felt I did not recognize my family. I was in my twenties when lupus struck, and now I was in my forties. My children had been raised by whoever was willing to help when I was sick. My business was gone. My home was lost. And the photos of me on the verge of death tainted my memories of that time. This was not the memory of the family I'd had before I got sick. I thought like a twenty-something but looked twice her age. That was when I realized I would have to learn how to be a mother and wife again.

My life would have been different if I had received the stem cell transplant when it was first offered. The possibility of not experiencing a heart attack, fibrosis, and kidney failure would have been substantial. In fact, I might have avoided most of the health problems I struggle with today—high blood pressure, colitis, shortness of breath, fatigue, and bone degeneration. The six-plus years of litigation and battling corruption at the highest levels would not have been necessary.

The Affordable Care Act split the country in two. Some thought it was too much too soon, while others believed it was not enough. I did hope it would set in place protections that limit situations like the one I lived through for almost a decade. Years later, the more things change, the more they stay the same. People are unsatisfied with the health insurance industry, politicians, and the lack of affordable health care.

I guess I'm one of the lucky ones. Many diagnosed with lupus survive only five to ten years. Dr. Burt's research team was vital to patient survival. Meeting Dr. Burt and working with the staff at Northwestern is something I do not regret, although I wish it had been under better circumstances. I wish I could see them all again to express my gratitude.

www.ingramcontent.com/pod-product-compliance
Lightning Source LLC
Chambersburg PA
CBHW020327170426
43200CB00006B/301